How's

Your

Marriage?

A Book for
Men and Women

How's

Your

Marriage?

A Book for
Men and Women

Michael F. Myers, M.D.

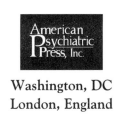

Washington, DC
London, England

Copyright © 1998 American Psychiatric Press, Inc.
ALL RIGHTS RESERVED
Manufactured in the United States of America on acid-free paper
First Edition
01 00 99 98   4 3 2 1
American Psychiatric Press, Inc.
1400 K Street, N.W., Washington, DC   20005
www.appi.org

Library of Congress Cataloging-in-Publication Data
Myers, Michael F.
    How's your marriage? : a book for men and women / Michael F. Myers.
        p.   cm.
    Includes bibliographical references and index.
    ISBN 0-88048-695-3
    1. Marriage.   2. Marital conflict.   3. Marital psychotherapy.
    4. Married people—Psychology.   I. Title.
HQ734.M986   1998
306.81—dc21   97-25511
                                                                 CIP

British Library Cataloguing in Publication Data
A CIP record is available from the British Library.

To Joice

Contents

Acknowledgments

want to thank Dr. Carol Nadelson for inviting me to write this book. I credit her with the vision of publishing a trade book on marriage authored by a psychiatrist. From the beginning, she has been my ballast. I cherish her steady support and our long friendship. My patients are my teachers, and I thank them for their wisdom. Thirty years of treating couples have taught me an enormous amount about the mysteries of marriage, the challenges of communication, the highs and the lows, and in the end, the resiliency of the human spirit. I continue to learn as I continue my work. I am indebted to my patients for their trust in me—and for the opportunity to enter the privacy of their relationships and families. My students are also my teachers. I could not have produced this book without their questions, hunches, and insights. Many have been there on the front lines, working alongside me as cotherapists. They continue to enrich my perspective and therapy. I thank them for their compassion for couples in distress, their empathic curiosity, and their willingness to help in any, and all, ways. Marilyn Weller, my editorial consultant, worked closely with me for months. I thank her for making many of the book's structural changes, for helping to eliminate the redundancy, and for making my prose less academic and more user-friendly. Most important, she made me laugh. Many others have helped enormously. Claire Reinberg, Editorial Director of American Psychiatric Press, Inc., has been there since the beginning. Her quiet and gentle support has been exceptional. Pamela Harley, Mark Bloom, Martin Lynds, and other APPI staff have given the book polish. I am grateful to all of them. Finally, I thank my wife Joice, my daughter Briana, and my son Zachary. I could not study and practice psychiatry and marital therapy without their love, commitment, expressiveness, and good humor. These values nurture and sustain our ever-evolving family journey.

Michael F. Myers, M.D.
Vancouver, British Columbia

Introduction

"Did you talk with Bart and Annette at the party tonight? They sure haven't looked very happy lately."

"I had lunch with Carol today. She and Jim are seeing a marriage counselor. Finally."

"Now I know why we haven't seen much of Ann and David the last few months. He's been having an affair with someone at work. We got into a few beers tonight and he told me."

"Joshua came home from school today and told me that Daniel's parents have split up. What a shock! They looked so happy at Sports Day."

"I feel so miserable, so empty, so lonely. And Thursday is our 25th wedding anniversary. I just want to run away."

Marital problems have reached epidemic proportions in North America. This is reflected in the number of couples who seek marital therapy each year, the number of individuals who visit their primary care physician with physical or emotional symptoms related to marital distress, the number of individuals who request personal psychotherapy because of marital concerns, the number of battered women seeking help, the number of battering husbands being arrested, and the vast number of separations and divorces each year.

I am a clinician who looks after people with troubled marriages. After completing medical school, internship, and a 4-year residency in general psychiatry, I accepted a half-time faculty position teaching medical students and residents and opened up a half-time private practice in adult psychiatry. This was in 1973. I was immediately struck by how many patients I was seeing for various psychiatric troubles who had marital (or relationship) problems. My head spun with questions: Is this person depressed because of a bad marriage? Is the marriage strained because the person is so ill, so unable to function, to contribute, to communicate, to laugh, to love? Or is this some complex reverberating circuit, with both my patient and his or her marriage caught up in a negative, downward, ever accelerating spiral? Might I possibly make things worse using conventional psychiatric methods, including well-intentioned psychotherapy? Might I be keeping this individual mired in a poor marriage with my treatment? Or the opposite, contributing to marriage breakdown, especially unnecessary breakdown, with my therapy?

Although I was versed in an eclectic understanding of the biological, psychological, and sociocultural underpinnings of psychiatric illness, the conventional approach was largely one-on-one—that is, individual therapy with "the patient." This seemed limiting and not helpful with many of my patients. So I decided to "do" couple therapy with them and their partners or spouses. And I signed up for more training in this field.

This period corresponded with the resurgence of the women's movement and the phenomenon of rapidly changing roles for women and men in marriage. More and more women were remaining in, or entering, the paid workforce after marriage and children, more and more marriages were becoming dual career or dual earner, and more and more couples were striving to share child care and domestic labor. I became fascinated by women's studies, and later men's studies, and what this research was telling us about the everyday lives of people in relationships: their differing expectations and new values, their frustrations and problems, and their symptoms, and how all of this was applicable to my daily work. This was a challenging and fruitful period in my professional and personal development as a man, as a psychiatrist, and as a marital therapist.

This book is the product of my 21 years of assessing couples and treating them with couple therapy. Although I usually refer to married couples, my experience is with a much larger group—couples who are not married but who are cohabiting; couples who are committed to each other but are not living together or married; couples who are married but living apart; couples who are divorced from each other (and perhaps are remarried to other people) but who come for couple therapy regarding their children; gay male couples; and lesbian couples. Hence, I hope that my observations and suggestions will be of help to a large group of people, not just people with troubled marriages.

This is a book for women and men. I have written from a gender perspective because so many problems in relationships are rooted in differing perceptions and misunderstandings: simply because he is a man and she is a woman, and what both of them bring from their personal, family, and social pasts into their relationship. The text is interspersed with disguised verbatim quotes from women and men in my practice—complaints that men make about their wives, that women make about their husbands. They are complaints uttered at one time by most couples. I try to explain some of the feelings and thoughts that surround these complaints and to offer solutions.

Because complaints about communication are ubiquitous, not just in couples who would define their relationship as stressed, I have devoted Chapter One to this matter. Why is it so hard to communicate effectively in marriage? How significant is our upbringing in how we communicate? Do men and women communicate differently? These are some of the questions that I put forward. The body of this chapter is composed of examples of couples with communication frustrations and my suggestions to them. I conclude with some lists: lists of common communication blocks, guidelines for more efficient conversation, and tips for fair fighting.

In Chapter Two I discuss how marriages have cycles and the relationship of these cycles to the life cycles through which all individuals must pass. I pose questions that men and women ask at various stages of marriage and I attempt to answer them—if not answer, then perhaps understand the "why" of the question. These serve to illustrate how much our thoughts, feelings, hopes, and dreams are colored by the cycles and stages in our lives and how these passages are different in many ways for women and for men.

Chapter Three on sexual problems in relationships is an overview of the most common types of sexual concerns in troubled marriages. I focus on the intricate relationship between marriage functioning and sexual functioning and describe in some detail the most common factors in a relationship that can affect sexual interest, frequency, and satisfaction. Once again, I point out some of the differences and similarities between women and men regarding their sexual wishes, needs, doubts, and pleasures.

Extramarital relationships almost always cause marital upset. They represent a threat, if not an assault, to marital integrity. Or if the marriage foundation was already a bit cracked, they can aggravate it—an earth tremor becomes an earthquake. I discuss extramarital relationships in some detail in Chapter Four: whether they are disclosed or "found out," what causes a man or woman to get involved with someone else, how this in turn affects one's spouse or partner, and what happens to the marriage in the short and long term.

"My husband (or wife) drinks too much." This is one of the most common complaints in unhappy marriages and, left untreated, causes heartache throughout the entire family. In Chapter Five, I describe the various kinds of drinking patterns in individuals (there are many) and how excessive alcohol affects marital communication, trust, sex, and solidarity. I have included here several clinical examples from my practice, what causes problem drinking, how you can tell if you or your spouse/partner is drinking too much, what to expect from your doctor, and what resources are available for you and your family.

In Chapter Six, "Psychiatric Illness and Marriage," I describe the two-way street that characterizes the relationship between one's mental health and one's marriage: how having a psychiatric illness affects marital function and how marital dysfunction affects mental health. I am quite emphatic in this chapter because the results can be disastrous if a mistake is made (e.g., the marriage gets treated when it's the individual who needs treatment or vice versa). I have seen too many people leave healthy marriages because they mistakenly concluded (as did their therapist) that the marriage was dead. And conversely, I have seen many individuals remain in toxic relationships because they mistakenly concluded (as did their therapist) that it was all their problem, that they were weak and "neurotic" and a loser, whereas their husband or wife was the paragon of mental health. Half this chapter is devoted to questions and answers about five psychiatric illnesses and their relationship to marriage: depression, panic disorder, agoraphobia, bipolar illness, and eating disorders.

In Chapter Seven, "The Role of Children in Marital Disharmony," I discuss the relationship between marital functioning and children. Not just how marital tension and unhappiness affect children but also how worry about and disappointments with children affect marriage. The relationship can indeed be very complex and confusing. Using case examples, I have given suggestions about what to do and how to get help. Included here is a section on stepfamilies and their struggles.

"What About Separation and Divorce?" is the title of Chapter Eight, and I hope that my comments help to diminish the reader's anxiety about what the outcome is for at least some people with marital concerns. A book about marriage is not complete without some discussion about separation and divorce.

The remaining chapters in this book are full of questions, explanations, and practical tips. Chapter Nine, "What You Can Do to Help Yourselves," is intended to be consciousness raising and alarm sounding: that you must pay attention to the warning signs of trouble or possible trouble, and that there is a lot that can be done early and preventively, if you like. Once again I illustrate many of my points with examples from my practice. People have an enormous number of questions and often a lot of anxiety (understandably so) about marital therapy and I try to answer all of them in the final three chapters. How does it work? Whom should we see? Should we see a man or a woman? What kinds of professionals do marital therapy? What should we expect? How long does it take? How do I get my spouse to go with me? And so forth.

I hope that this book captures the perspective, and the interest, that I bring to my daily work with couples. It is a physicianly vision of emotional pain and loneliness in relationships, of fear and inhibition, xvi How's Your Marriage? A Book for Men and Women

of courage and confrontation, of hope and renewal. I have tried to produce a volume that both enlightens and guides, a book that speaks to some of the conflict and unhappiness of people's lives today and what to do about it. My case illustrations are all composites from my practice and are deliberately altered to protect my patients' identities and to preserve their confidentiality.

ONE

Communication

Good communication is central to healthy relationships. "We're not communicating very well" is one of the most common and frustrating concerns couples experience. It is normal for a couple to have occasional communication problems. But when these problems happen frequently, it is a serious matter that needs attention.

To say that we're not communicating very well with our spouse can mean many different things. There is usually a sense that what we are trying to say is not being received very well, or even listened to, judging by our spouse's response or lack of response. What we then tend to do is jump to conclusions about our spouse, without checking out what he or she heard us say. We attribute motives to our spouse that are not accurate or even true, then we react to how he or she has responded. Very soon the original statement or message is completely lost. This kind of communication often produces tension, arguing, defensiveness, exasperation, and withdrawal or silence in one or the other.

Another common problem is that to some people, not communicating may mean not talking at all, or not talking enough. At least one of the two individuals then feels frustrated, angry, sad, or lonely.

Very often, as is discussed later in this chapter, this is the woman in the marriage. This difference is very common in marriage and many people simply adapt. It becomes a problem when it occurs often or arises for no obvious reason.

"We're not communicating" can also mean "We're too busy to talk" or "We don't set aside time to talk." This isn't uncommon in the 1990s, with couples leading fast-paced lives and with so many marriages in which both partners are working outside the home. The implication is "If we only had time to talk, we could communicate well about issues." This assumption may or may not be true because their communication ability hasn't actually been tested.

When only one partner is complaining about communication, sometimes he or she means "We can only talk about superficial or 'safe' subjects." There is a concern that deep and possibly upsetting matters never get discussed and are glossed over for fear of upsetting a rather shaky or tenuous equilibrium. If a partner takes pride in his or her communication abilities, this complaint can sound insulting.

Women often identify and air concerns about change in marital

---

He Says . . .

"She works too hard. But when I say anything, she gets defensive and says I'm trying to control her."

It has only been in the last few decades that more and more women have been in the paid workforce for most of their adult lives. It is also only a relatively short time since large numbers of women began pursuing careers or since wanting a career became "normal" and to be expected. Dual-paycheck couples are much more common than single-earner couples nowadays. But this has not changed many attitudes and expectations about men's and women's roles.

Most of the married women with children who are working outside the home are doing it for a number of reasons. Sometimes it is simple economic necessity. But there is a large group of women who want to work outside the home. Their work meets many of their personal needs for accomplishment, intellectual stimulation, fulfillment, challenge, relationships, and economic independence.

It is easy to see, then, why some women become defensive when they are criticized or attacked by their husbands for working too hard. What gets missed in the discussion is not so much that she is working outside the home but how much. And why her husband is complaining is not so often a control issue (although in some marriages it is) but one of unmet needs—his! What he is not saying is that he is feeling lonely in his marriage.

communication long before their husbands. Through the years, women have done the "worry work" of marriage; that is, they have tended to the health of their marriage in much the same way they have tended to their children, their homes, and their communities. For the past two decades, with changing gender roles affecting marital dynamics in many different ways, more men are beginning to have concerns about communication in their marriage, perhaps because of a decline in the stigma associated with recognizing communication problems in relationships and reaching out for professional help.

Why Is It So Hard to Communicate in Relationships?

None of us are born with an innate ability to communicate easily. However, if you grow up in a home where open and direct communication among family members is present, then you have an advantage in understanding how to talk with others outside your family. What is essential is a desire and willingness to communicate effectively in love relationships, fully knowing that this means taking risks, revealing painful or embarrassing things about yourself, and knowing that you will hear upsetting things said to you from time to time by your spouse or partner.

People vary enormously in their ability to know what their needs are and to communicate them clearly. Clifford Sager, a psychiatrist and marital therapist, believes that there are three different levels of communication in marriage: *conscious and verbalized, conscious but not verbalized,* and *beyond awareness.*

When we communicate at a *conscious and verbalized* level, we talk about matters that we are aware of and have no difficulty expressing to our spouse. This is easy, straightforward, and usually goal oriented and problem solving so we feel listened to and understood. There is a sense of comfort, achievement, and solidarity when the bulk of communication is like this. This is the clearest and most direct form of communication.

Conscious but not verbalized communication is more complicated.

One or both of the marriage partners are aware of thoughts and feelings that they do not express. Why not? There are many reasons. The individual may never have been very open or communicative. He or she may be a quiet, shy, or private person. Perhaps he or she was raised in a home atmosphere that was not very expressive, or he or she may have been criticized, scolded, or beaten for expressing feelings or opinions. Some people in marriage monitor or censor what they say because they have perceived or learned over the course of their relationship that some subjects precipitate strong emotions (crying, hurt, sadness, rage, guilt, anxiety) or frightening behavior (verbal retaliation, physical violence, sexual forcefulness, drinking, silent withdrawal, abandonment) in their spouse. Consequently, many issues never get talked about and communication stays at a very superficial, polite, or prosaic level.

Beyond awareness is complicated because it contains the conflicts of which we are not even aware, and therefore we can't discuss them. Because the conflicts are unconscious, we may get glimpses or fragments from our dreams—not always the actual content that we recall on awakening but certainly the themes or mood of our dreams, fantasies, or feelings. We may have a dream of being the perpetrator or victim of aggression, being lost, running away, feeling controlled or trapped, or being sexually or emotionally involved with someone other than our partner. We may also get clues of unconscious and unexpressed feelings and ideas when we've had too much to drink and we lose our inhibitions and say things or behave in certain ways that would not occur otherwise. Sarcasm is often indicative of unconscious hostility toward our partner and we may not be aware of it until we hear ourselves speak or are called on it.

Mr. and Mrs. M came for therapy saying, "We have major problems with communication. We can't discuss the weather without arguing." In their early visits I was struck by the degree of verbal competition that existed between them. They argued about almost everything. Although they complained about this, I was aware that they also enjoyed the verbal games they played with each other. Their respective vocabularies were dazzling and I struggled not to get caught up in the intellectual volley. They were both very bright and skilled at holding their own in the minefield of marital communication.

My individual interviews with each of them had yielded important information that they were not sharing or had not shared with each other. For example, Mr. M's first girlfriend in high school became pregnant by him and had an abortion, about which he felt guilty and ashamed. He had had a psychotic experience, possibly drug induced, when he traveled abroad while in college. Mrs. M had also had an abortion in the past and had told no one except a close woman friend. She had cheated once on a very important exam, and, although she was never found out, she ruminated about this from time to time in a guilty and remorseful way. I wondered if much of their verbal sparring was a defense against a deeper level of communication and vulnerability. I floated this hunch before them in one particularly tense visit and asked each of them to consider disclosing some of the many feelings that they had discussed with me privately.

What followed was an exciting period of several weeks where they talked more openly and deeply than they had ever done. They felt much closer, they were certainly more affectionate with each other in my office, and they noted that their sexual relationship had become more passionate and interesting. Their arguing was less frequent and less volatile.

After several conjoint visits, Mr. M announced that he had something quite frightening and embarrassing to bring up. He had had a dream about 5 days previously from which he awakened in a cold sweat. Just before awakening, he remembered touching the penis of a 9-year-old boy. He was mortified and couldn't go back to sleep. He hadn't told his wife about the dream until recounting it in her presence in my office. She was very comforting and reassuring as he tearfully wondered aloud, "What does this mean? Am I gay? Am I a pedophile?" I asked him if anyone had ever touched him in a similar way when he was a boy. He said "no" very quickly and then said, "Wait a minute!" and began to cry. After a few minutes he recalled being fondled by a priest after assisting with mass as an altar boy when he was "about 8 or 9." Mrs. M spontaneously said, "I think I know why you hate me to stimulate your penis with my hand during foreplay."

This vignette, greatly condensed, describes how communication at a conscious and verbalized level was not clear and certainly not adequate for this highly functioning couple. Communication at a conscious but previously nonverbalized level led to a sense of relief, common purpose, problem solving, and enhanced intimacy. Communication at a previously unconscious level led to even more understanding and mutual sensitivity.

What You Were Taught

To understand more fully the difficulties in marital communication, it helps to think about childhood and family dynamics, especially the marriage or marriages of your parents. Whether we like it or not, our parents are the first, if not only, role models we are exposed to in terms of how two adults communicate in a love relationship. Think how complex that is for people today! In a room of 10 adults, here are 10 possibilities: someone raised by two parents in a reasonably happy marriage that lasted 45 years until one of them died; someone whose parents divorced when he was 10 years old, his father remarried within 2 years, his mother never remarried and remained bitter the rest of her life; someone raised by a single mother who was never married, she never knew her father; someone whose parents divorced when she was 6 years old, her father remarried and divorced twice more, her mother remarried only once but lives in a very unhappy second marriage; someone whose mother died when he was 11 years old and whose father never dated again or remarried; someone who grew up in a series of foster homes, living in none of them for more than 2 years; someone who was conceived by artificial insemination and whose mother has been in a stable lesbian relationship for over 30 years; someone who has grown up in a joint custody arrangement since the age of 4, 1 week at Dad's home, 1 week at Mom's; someone whose father was at sea in the merchant marines and was home only a few months a year; and someone who was sent away to boarding school at age 7 and really only saw his parents over Christmas break and summer vacation. These situations illustrate that there is an enormous range of adult figures who may influence, for better or for worse, how a child learns to communicate his or her thoughts and feelings.

But our ability to communicate in marriage is not only dependent on what we've learned from parents or parent figures; it also can have a genetic component. For example, if my biological father suffered from schizophrenia and had a severe disturbance in his ability to think and to speak, I may have an inherited tendency to be at risk myself for the same disorder, even if my adoptive parents had a perfect marriage and were my role models since I was a baby. Or if my mother suffered repeated severe depressions wherein she withdrew to her room for days on end and didn't speak, I may be at risk myself to "shut down" verbally, not just because I learned it from her but because I'm genetically prone to depression myself.

With the above in mind, when appropriate it is a good idea to ask yourself some of the following questions:

- What are the similarities and the differences between my marriage and my parents' marriage or marriages?
- In what ways am I like my mother in how I communicate, in what ways like my father?
- Do my parents express feelings much when they talk to each other?
- Is there a difference between the two of them in emotional expressiveness?
- How affectionate were the two of them toward each other when I was growing up, both in words (terms of endearment) and in action (hugs, kisses, holding hands)?
- Did they argue or fight much?
- How did my parents handle stress?

These questions have as their goal insight and change. They arise from a developmental premise that all of us are shaped by a mix of biological, psychological, social, cultural, political, and economic factors that we bring into our marriages. These determine our needs, attitudes, values, and expectations. These questions, and many others, are directed at the self, and that's important because until we can ask them courageously and honestly, it is very hard, if not impossible, to communicate maturely and constructively in our marriages.

Men and Women
Communicate Differently

This is a big subject and one about which volumes of research have been conducted over the past decade. I will highlight some of the more relevant results and conclusions.

Men tend not to be as aware of their feelings as women. Their feelings are more likely to be hidden, not only from themselves but from their wives and others. Hence they may appear on the surface to be less reactive, cooler, calmer, more self-contained, and private. As a result many women describe feeling lonely in their marriages. They complain either that their husbands don't talk to them enough or that their husbands don't share inner and personal thoughts and emotions. In fact, many women complain that they are forever "second-guessing" or "reading between the lines" with their partners. This difference between men and women is probably constitutional—it just *is*. It does not mean that one gender is better than the other, or that one is normal and the other is not.

Let me emphasize something here. Men who don't talk much may still be communicating a great deal to their wives. They communicate a lot by their silence, by being absent or withdrawn, by overworking, by holding back their feelings, by drinking, by making repeated and unwelcome sexual demands, and by their aggressive posturing or violent acts. These are all forms of communication, albeit oblique, inappropriate, and confusing. Tremendous power and control are contained in these behaviors, which are destructive to their wives' self-worth and safety and toxic to marital harmony and intimacy.

Deborah Tannen, author of *You Just Don't Understand: Women and Men in Conversation* and professor of linguistics at Georgetown University, has studied differing conversational styles in men and women. She believes that friction arises because boys and girls grow up in what are essentially different cultures, so that talk between women and men is cross-cultural communication. Her observations of asymmetries in speech, interruptions in conversation, gossip, and silence are splendid and go a long way toward reassuring men and women in marriage that they are not crazy or wrong, just different.

Examples of Communication Problems

Because men and women are so different in their attitudes, conversational styles, and willingness to talk to each other, they are prone to misunderstandings and communication failures on many subjects: money, sex, children, their respective families, work, friends, and domestic responsibilities. What follows are snippets about some couples and their communication concerns. These examples are not complete in any sense of the word, and the suggestions I discuss are meant to be merely illustrative of simple interventions. They do not capture the duration or the intensity of marital therapy.

Tom and Janice

The first words out of Janice's mouth when she and Tom came to see me were "If we don't get some help, we're not going to make it." She continued in an angry, desperate way for a few minutes more. Some of what she said was "I've had it. Tom's a workaholic and he seems to be getting worse the more successful he becomes. He sees me as a complaining bitch, and he's right, I'm always angry now and sarcastic when he's around. Our problem is so simple: we don't spend enough time together. I'm so lonely I could scream."

While Janice spoke, Tom kept interrupting and gesturing wildly in apparent disbelief or outrage about her complaints. He looked out the window and shook his head. He looked at me and rolled his eyes. He'd glance at her with a look of rage or disdain.

Finally, I gently cut in and asked Tom to present his concerns about their marriage. He began in an angry, defensive, attacking, and long-winded way (I had to eventually interrupt him too): "Don't listen to what she's saying. Her reality is not my reality. I'm not a workaholic, not as I would define it, and I don't work like 90% of the men I know. Janice has never been happy a day in her life; even her mother said she scowled in the delivery room the day she was born. We don't have a marital problem, Janice has a problem, a long-standing one, it's called a problem with life. I don't have time for this. I should be at my office right now, doing what's important in life."

I knew I had my work cut out for me with Tom and Janice! They both felt unhappy, demoralized, misunderstood by the other, and uncertain whether marital therapy could help.

Suggestions

1. "Listen; don't interrupt."
2. "Start from a clean slate despite unhappiness and a lot of water under the bridge."
3. "Watch the 'absolutes' (never, always, etc.)."
4. "Try to remain hopeful that talking to a professional can help."

Rita and Sam

In their initial visit, Rita spoke first: "I want marital therapy because I've been going through a lot of changes, I've grown in many ways, and this has affected our marriage. I've been in treatment for 2 years with another psychiatrist for my bulimia. I'm a lot stronger now and in more control of my problem. But now I want to work on our marriage."

Sam responded with "I'm here because I'm worried about money. My wife spends too much; she's going to drive us into the poorhouse—we can't discuss it—all we do is argue."

Other facts emerged from the first visit. Sam had bought his own business after many years as a laborer and they were trying to live on a very tight budget, which was formidable and depressing for Rita. They came from different socioeconomic backgrounds: Sam from a struggling single-parent family, Rita from a comfortable middle-class family. Rita had been epileptic since age 15, a real challenge for her. In addition, they were an infertile couple and were foster parents for Sam's niece, a situation to which they were adjusting. All considered, they were coping with a lot of disappointments and stresses in their lives.

Suggestions

1. "Get some control over credit card expenditures."
2. "Redo the budget—make provision for a bit more spending money and funds for a 'date' together at least once every 2 weeks."
3. To Rita: "Be more direct and honest with your concerns about Sam's controlling nature and your own responsive behaviors."

4. To Sam: "Watch your 'parent' role with Rita and speak as adult to adult, not parent to child."

Betty and David

This couple couldn't have sat farther apart from each other in my office. Both of them looked very sad and "beaten down." David started first: "I had an affair; it's killing Betty." Betty cut in: "Had? What about, 'I'm having an affair'? I think that would be more accurate." Silence.

David started again: "I met another woman, we got sexually involved, it's sort of over, I think." More silence. I asked Betty how all of this had been for her. She stated, "Well, he's right, this is killing me. I can't sleep, I can't eat, I've lost 10 pounds in 10 days, I can't stop crying, and I can't stop hating him."

She continued: "I'm furious, I'm jealous, and I'm scared stiff. I don't want to be on my own at 50. Our kids are in university and more or less grown up." Turning to David, she said, "Thanks for dumping me when I don't serve any purpose anymore."

He looked away, angrily, and then looked at me, his eyes filling with tears: "I only got involved with Mona because I felt Betty despised me. She hasn't said one encouraging thing to me in 5 years, mainly since my business went belly-up. I've felt like such a loser in the workforce and a loser at home too. I never knew how lonely I was until Mona started paying attention to me, and it built from there. I'm really confused now. Even though Betty hates me, she says she also loves me. I didn't know that before."

Suggestions

1. "Don't make any decisions yet about the marriage. Give marital therapy a chance over the next month to 6 weeks."
2. "David, you must end the relationship with Mona if you intend to work on your marriage. Think about it. You can't do both. If you decide to continue to see Mona, that you love her and can't give her up, and if you, Betty, would want to separate, then I'll help you both with that if you want my assistance."
3. "Keep talking but take time out if it gets too tense, hostile, and there is too much mudslinging."
4. In my individual sessions with each of them, I would be especially

careful to assess Betty for depression and would treat accordingly if necessary.

5. "Acknowledge that there is no trust, or very little, at present. If the marriage is salvageable, it will take a while for trust to be regained."
6. "Try your best to reassure each other when you can, when you feel positive about your feelings, when you feel hopeful."
7. "Try to talk about the feeling that you *both* are experiencing of being unlovable."
8. "Give time a chance. In situations like this, time is the best healer. And over time things will become much clearer regarding your lives, whether you remain together, happily, as a couple, or whether you separate."

Bill and Dennis

Bill and Dennis were gay and both had AIDS. They had been together for 5 years, having met each other in a support group for people with AIDS. This was their first serious, committed relationship. When they initially came for treatment, my work with them was largely focused on their adjustment to moving in together and to living with profound loss. They were both medically stable, working full time, and, with limitations, enjoying their lives together and with their friends.

I had not seen them for nearly 3 years when they again came from the hospital AIDS clinic to my office. They were in a serious crisis. Bill, who had originally been much less ill than Dennis, was now living with very advanced AIDS, including losing his vision from CMV (cytomegaloviral) retinitis. This had been devastating for Dennis, who had become quite depressed and returned to using heroin. This, in turn, disgusted Bill, whose father, once a successful attorney, died homeless, an incorrigible alcoholic. Bill was furious at Dennis for not being "strong."

Suggestions

1. To Dennis: "I have to admit you to detox. You've only been back on heroin briefly and you should do fine. After a week, you'll go for a month of residential care. They will watch your mood there and put you back on medication if you get depressed."
2. To Bill: "I'd like you to start going to Narcanon, a step program for partners and spouses of people who are addicted to drugs."

3. To Bill (after Dennis returned from residential treatment and they came to a session together): "Try to talk to Dennis about your feelings about dying and how much you need his support."

4. To Dennis (in another conjoint visit): "Let's talk about your 'slip' back into taking drugs. Is it about despair and frustration living with AIDS? About pain, grief, stigmatization? About loneliness and losing Bill?"

5. To both: "How about returning to some low-key social activities together? Perhaps you could take walks together in the park or trips to the beach? These outings might help you both to talk more openly and share your time together."

Connie and Hank

This couple's concerns were with two of their three young adult sons who were still living at home. One of them had been unemployed for 6 months, had no friends, and slept and watched TV most of the time. (By Connie's description, he seemed depressed.) The other was going to college part-time and working, but he spent most of his free time drinking. Given the numbers of relatives on both sides who were alcoholic, their worries seemed valid, but Connie and Hank could not discuss many important matters, including these two children.

This situation was extremely frustrating for Connie, and this was why she wanted Hank to come with her for marital therapy. "I just want to be heard. Hank's detachment, his denial of any problems at home, and his obsession with his work and his sports are driving me nuts." Hank looked at her with a big grin on his face and then he turned to me: "Connie's a worrywart. I just whistle and smile and go about my business. I read Norman Vincent Peale's *The Power of Positive Thinking* in high school and it's never failed me since."

Suggestions

1. "Make time at least twice a week to go out together, even if it's just for a walk. My sense is that the two of you are not spending enough one-on-one time with each other. Your lives are both very busy."

2. "Use this time, when you're not at home, to talk about your sons."

3. To Connie: "Ask for support and dialogue at the time rather than letting things build up and becoming anxious about everything."

4. To Hank: "You must listen and stop sweeping family issues under

the carpet. The philosophy of life that works for you isn't working for the two of you. You can't ignore possible problems with your sons, despite the fact that they are now adults. They do live in your home, must follow house rules, and still probably need your guidance and wisdom."

5. "Insist that both sons talk to professionals, for an assessment of their mental health and chemical dependency. Approach them warmly yet firmly. They must also be expected to take some part in the running of the home. They are not merely boarders or freeloaders. Even if they are diagnosed with a psychiatric illness, they can take part in making your house a home."

6. To Hank: "Try to open up a bit more about yourself. Despite your positive attitude, there must be times when you feel a bit down or frightened. If you share those moments with Connie, I think she will find you more real. Try to be more reassuring to Connie and not so judgmental when she's feeling anxious. Until your sons are more functional, she has every reason, as a caring parent, to be worried."

John and Jane

This couple's main concern about their marriage was "sex," namely that Jane had lost all interest in sex since their son Adrian was born. He was now 3 years old. Jane was certain that something had happened to her while giving birth to Adrian, that she had been damaged in some way. I asked more specifically about this and learned that her labor and delivery had been quite straightforward. She delivered Adrian vaginally with very little medication, no episiotomy, and no tears or lacerations. She had been examined by two gynecologists about her sexual concerns before seeing me and neither could find anything wrong physically. Her general physical health was fine.

John was angry toward and critical of Jane for her lack of interest in sex. He wondered if the problem was her diet and thought she should become a vegetarian. He insisted, though, on "sex therapy" because he felt that Jane was "abnormal" and should be "fixed."

What I noticed about Jane and John was that they were both preoccupied with their sexual problem to the exclusion of everything else in their relationship. Further, they talked about sex in a very mechanistic and impersonal manner, almost as if they were struggling with a broken instrument or vehicle that needed to be repaired. Neither used emotional language (except frustration at the problem).

In my individual visits with each of them I learned a lot about their backgrounds, which had been very painful (divorces by their parents, violence, murder of a twin sister, death of a brother by suicide, and severe poverty). Both had coped by being strong, forward thinking, and deeply religious.

Current stressors in their lives were the following: financial troubles (even though they both worked full-time, money was tight); John was drinking quite a bit (even though neither thought it was a problem, I certainly did!); Jane was really tired working full-time and being a mother and homemaker (John was not very helpful at home and once again I thought this was more of a problem than either of them did); and both were worried about ADHD (attention-deficit/hyperactivity disorder) in their older son Brad, who was having numerous learning and behavioral problems at school.

Suggestions

1. To both: "Don't discuss sex! Your sexual problem is a relationship problem. This will become clearer with more sessions. There is nothing wrong with your sexuality, Jane. You do not need to be 'fixed.'"
2. "Work on increasing physical affection with each other and verbal gestures of fondness and loving."
3. "Spend some time alone as a couple."
4. To Jane: "Begin to talk to John directly about your concerns and complaints in the marriage."
5. To John: "Specifically ask Jane for compliments and affection until all of this comes a bit more naturally. Also think about one of the meanings of sex to you, that is, that being sexual together reduces your feelings of insecurity and fears that you will be abandoned by Jane. (John's mother had "run off" with another man when he was 8 years old; John's first wife had ended their marriage and moved away, making him suspicious that she had found another man elsewhere.)
6. To both: "If things go well in our visits together, and your marriage improves, I expect your sex life to return to normal or to become better than normal."

Elsie and Clyde

Elsie and Clyde were a couple in their mid-50s. Their chief complaint was "We're bored with each other and don't know whether to stay together or not." Their three children had grown, were all married, and were living on their own. Elsie had not worked outside the home since before she was married. She especially felt lonely married to Clyde, who was busy with his job as a bus driver, with golf, and with church activities. They occasionally went out with friends but "never did anything" as a couple, and they sat in silence most of the time at meals or while driving in the car. My assessment of the two of them and their marriage did not reveal any deep-seated psychological or psychiatric problems in either of them or their families.

Suggestions

1. "Go for walks together on a regular basis."
2. "Sign up for a marital enrichment weekend through your church."
3. "Read to each other. Take turns reading essays, short stories, or poetry aloud."
4. To Clyde: "What would you do this weekend with Elsie if you had just met and you were interested in having a date with her?" This question made him laugh and also blush. He hesitated, then said he'd like to go dancing, just like they did on their first date almost 30 years earlier. Touched, Elsie's eyes filled with tears.
5. To Elsie: "If you could ask any question of Clyde and get an honest answer, what would it be?" She reflected, then asked him, "Do you really love me? I get the feeling you're bored with me." He hesitated and said, "I do love you, I really do; but you're right, I do get bored when we're together. You talk about stuff that doesn't interest me, and I just blank out. I start daydreaming about fishing." Elsie admitted that Clyde was so quiet and not talkative so she tended to fill in silences with talk about superficial topics. "I hate the quietness, it's like cancer, like a death," she said.
6. To both: "Brainstorm to find some hobbies, activities, interests, courses, or games that appeal to both of you, so you have some interests in common."
7. To Elsie: "How about taking up another interest or two of your own?"

Tina and Nick

This couple came for marital therapy with concerns that are common in blended families. Nick had been married before and had two children—Amy, 12, and Andrew, 9—who stayed with Tina and him every other weekend. Tina's words were "I really love Amy and Andrew; it's Nick who drives me nuts. He's so defensive of his kids, especially Amy, that I can't say one word about them or to them without Nick saying I'm too critical. Amy is being very difficult these days, she's 12 after all, but Nick expects me to just sit and not say a word. I'm getting really resentful."

Nick responded with "Tina's not being truthful. She doesn't love my kids; in fact, I think she can't stand them. She gets uptight as the time approaches for them to come and she's either ignoring them or making excuses to do things by herself when they're with us for the weekend. Amy has picked this up. She told me last time she doesn't want to come over to the house anymore because she thinks that Tina's mad at her. I think Tina's just jealous; I told her I was a 'package deal' on our first date, so she can't accuse me of not being straight with her."

Suggestions

1. To Nick: "You must begin to talk about your feelings of being caught in the middle between your kids and your wife, because my hunch is that you love and care about all of them. I want you to think about something: Do you feel guilty that your first marriage ended and you've had to put your kids through a divorce? If you do, that's normal. And if so, this might be why Tina finds you so defensive when the two of you try to discuss your kids."
2. To Tina: "You must begin to talk about your feelings of frustration, at times, about marrying a man who's a father and having to share him with his children. As you know, it's much simpler (not necessarily better) to marry a man who's not a father. Is Nick correct? Is it jealousy you feel or something else, like frustration or confusion?"
3. To Nick: "You must be more reassuring to Tina that you really do love her and want to be with her, that she and the children are equal priorities in your life and that you have no regrets about leaving your first wife."
4. To Tina: "Would you like more authority and responsibility for

Amy and Andrew? Do you find your role as a stepmother uncertain, restricted, or ambiguous? Perhaps you and Nick need to spend more time discussing this."

Brian and Mora

Brian and Mora were both 26 years old and graduate students. They had been living together for a year when they came to see me. Their complaint (which was largely emanating from Brian) was that they were not having sex very often. "I hate it. I bet my grandparents are getting it on more often than we are, and they're in their 70s."

Mora spoke next: "I was raped 2 years ago, and I met Brian shortly afterwards. Needless to say, it's been difficult (she begins to cry and Brian takes her hand). Brian thinks I'm obsessed with what happened to me and hates me to bring it up. I've been seeing a therapist ever since it happened, and that's been very helpful in my healing. I'm still in therapy because of stuff that I had buried, like abuse by my older brother when I was a little girl. And (turning to Brian) you hate my therapist, don't you? (Turning back to me) My therapist is a lesbian."

Suggestions

1. To Brian: "Read about sexual assault, especially the consequences for the victim and the victim's partner or spouse."
2. To Mora: "Continue in therapy as you've been doing and try to discuss the parts of it that you feel comfortable sharing with Brian."
3. To Brian: "Look at your feelings about the following questions: Are you having any concerns that Mora has come to fear or hate men in general as a result of being raped? Are you afraid that she'll become a lesbian and leave you? Are you afraid of your own feelings toward her assailant, like wanting to kill him? Is your infrequent sexual relationship with Mora affecting your sexual confidence as a man? It might help you to know that many young men equate infrequent sex with feelings of inadequacy."
4. To Mora: "What are some of your fears? Are you afraid that Brian might leave you (because you're not interested enough in sex, or that he perceives you as "damaged goods," or that he'll see you as a "bitch") if things don't get better soon? Are you afraid that you'll never get over the traumatic assault and feel whole again? Are you afraid of your relationships becoming like the lives of your parents

(both of Mora's parents had been married and divorced twice and were not very happy with their current lives)?"

Points to Consider

I hope that the previous series of vignettes has been helpful in illustrating some of the common types of communication problems in couples. As you can see, the issue of communication breakdown is both the "what" (the content) and the "how" (the process). What we talk about in our relationships dictates how we communicate. In general, the more painful or upsetting the subject is for the individual and/or the partner, the more difficult it is to discuss and the more confusing or blocked the communication patterns can become.

Blocks to Listening

Listening is critical in good communication. Seemingly simple, it is actually a very complex process that often goes awry when people, especially those in an intimate relationship, talk with each other. Here are some factors that cause a breakdown in listening and some processes that get in the way when we should be listening to what our spouse or partner is saying to us.

Comparing.   We are so busy comparing what he or she is saying to us or what others have said or might say that we really don't listen attentively. "You drink too much" prompts an immediate retort of "You eat too much!" or "Your father drinks a heck of a lot more than I do!"

Mind reading.   We are distracted from listening because we anticipate what our spouse is about to say or is really thinking or feeling but not saying aloud.

Rehearsing.   We can't listen because we are preparing our response. This is most likely to occur if we're feeling attacked or criticized. We begin to feel defensive and attack back with a criticism.

Filtering.   We only listen to certain things said to us.

Judging.   We can't listen effectively because we are critically ana-lyzing what our spouse is saying. There is a condemnatory tone to our response.

Dreaming.   We are not listening well because we are off somewhere in fantasy. We are daydreaming.

Identifying.   We may be identifying with what our spouse is saying and therefore respond with a similar experience that has happened to ourselves. In a sense, we negate what is special and unique about what's just been said to us. Further, we probably don't even ask our spouse to tell us more about it because we've already started to tell our own identical experience, as in the following: "(Interrupting) My boss does that to me too! Let me tell you what he did last week. . . ."

Advising.   This is very common in husbands in response to their wives talking about an upsetting experience at work, with a friend, with anyone. The man listens for a while, then begins to offer solu-tions. He finds himself upset when his wife is not interested in his sug-gestions. If she had asked him for advice in the first place, then that's a different matter. But most often she just wanted to ventilate about something that's bothering her and wants to feel listened to and sup-ported, not advised. Advising also has a dismissive connotation to it, implying "I've listened enough now, here's what to do, case closed."

Sparring.   This often occurs in couples who already have underly-ing marital struggles and who are not feeling very close to each other. There is an underlying sense of mistrust and power struggle. There-fore, their communication is marked by arguing, discounting of what's been said, debating almost every matter that's raised, and putting each other down.

Being right.   It is very frustrating when one spouse behaves or re-sponds as if he or she is always right. Rarely do people realize how arro-gant they sound or seem to be and how they use this as a way of not listening to what their spouses are saying. It is really a defense against admitting to oneself that you're as human and vulnerable as the next person.

Derailing. We derail a conversation when we suddenly change the subject. This blocks listening and usually means that what our spouse is saying isn't keeping our attention, that we're bored, or that we're so preoccupied with our own issues that we can't focus on anything else. It can also mean that what our spouse is saying is making us upset (nervous, sad, guilty, ashamed, angry, etc.), so we change the subject so we don't have to feel unpleasant emotions.

Placating. When we do this, we are agreeing seemingly whole-heartedly with what we're hearing but we are actually only partially listening. It is confusing for the person speaking, who believes that he or she has the other's undivided attention.

Effective Listening

I have four suggestions that go a long way toward helping us listen more effectively.

Listen actively. Paraphrase what your spouse or partner has just said. "Let me see if I understand what you just said to me. Are you saying that you . . . ?" Another way of listening actively is to clarify. Ask some questions to get more of the picture: "How old is he? Have you known him long? How'd you feel when you saw him?" A third form of active listening is to give some feedback to your spouse about what he or she has been saying: "I think you're feeling passed over at work. Is that so?"

Listen with empathy. In other words, try to put yourself in your spouse's shoes and experience what he or she is describing. "What does it feel like? Upsetting? Humiliating? Frightening?" Given your spouse's personality or emotional vulnerabilities (of which you are already aware), it should not be too hard for you to identify with what is being experienced. Your spouse, in turn, will feel that you are listening closely.

Listen with openness. Don't jump to conclusions in a habitual or knee-jerk manner. Wait until you've heard the whole story or statement. Try not to judge. This will be very hard to do at first if you are the type of person who normally finishes people's sentences and responds before they've finished what they were trying to say.

Listen with awareness. If you're having trouble paying attention, see if it's caused by external or internal interference. If it's external, try to do something about it: turn off the radio or TV, ask others to be quiet or move out of their area, ask your spouse to speak more slowly or more quickly, and so forth. If the problem is internal, tell your spouse that this isn't a good time to talk, that you're having trouble listening because you're tired, preoccupied, depressed, sick, or whatever the reason may be.

Guidelines for Good Communication

Here are some ideas that help to make talking to each other more productive and pleasurable.

- Prepare what you want to say, especially if it's something that's not easy to talk about. You may even want to write all or part of it down on paper so you can refer to it, or have your spouse read it if you like.
- Check to see that your spouse is in the mood to talk to you. Alert him or her if it's something quite serious or potentially upsetting.
- Use active listening (as described previously).
- Be as positive as possible. If it's a criticism of your spouse, put it in the form of a request rather than a complaint. For example, try "I'd like you to pick up your dirty clothes and put them in the hamper" rather than "You always leave your dirty clothes on the floor." Or, "Please don't tell the neighbors about my dad's affair" instead of "You've got a big mouth." Or, "I would really like you to come to

Parent Effectiveness Training with me. I think there's a lot about raising our kids that we can both learn from the experts" rather than "You yell at the kids one minute and spoil them the next."

- Use "I" messages. For example, "I'd really like you to take over the accounting at home. I'm not so good at it and I think you manage money better than I do." Or, "I'm really upset about what happened last night."
- Avoid "you" messages. For example, "You never tell me you love me" or "You're pretty controlling."
- Be specific. Only bring up what's concerning you right now. Give the exact example, not several or a generalization based on the example. "I felt you acted selfishly last night when I told you I was tired and you refused to leave the party until you had had another beer." As opposed to "I think you're selfish" or "You're so selfish."
- Stay focused. Don't bring up examples from 2 months ago or 2 years ago. Don't compare your spouse with his or her mother or father or with an idealized friend. For example, "You did the same thing on our honeymoon and that really hurt me. You're just like your father, very pigheaded. Why can't you be like Tom? He's so flexible and he never gets defensive like you."
- Agree to experiment for the next week or month with some new behavior. This applies to both of you. It won't work, nor is it fair, for one of you to be trying some new action when the other isn't. If you notice yourself slipping, apologize. Invite your spouse to gently remind you if you don't notice, and vice versa.
- Somehow acknowledge to your spouse that you really appreciate being able to talk about your concerns, even if it's a bit (or a lot!) upsetting. "I'm really pleased that you seem to feel like I do, that it's important to clear the air, that we need to let each other know if we're upset about something, and try to talk it through."

How to Fight Fair

- Don't threaten your spouse or partner.
- No name calling, like "You're a jerk."
- Stay on the topic being discussed.

- Don't interrupt. And don't go on and on so that your spouse has no choice but to interrupt. Be fair.
- Don't dominate by looking down at your spouse.
- Do not use absolutes like "never" or "always."
- Don't lecture.
- Take responsibility for your own feelings.
- Be prepared to change something about yourself.
- Don't blow the issue out of proportion.
- Let your spouse take time to reflect on what he or she is feeling.
- Try for a solution to the argument as opposed to some other motive.
- Don't attack verbally and certainly not physically. If things are getting out of hand, take time out from each other for 30 minutes to an hour and plan to talk later.
- Avoid dumping of stored-up hurts and resentments that go back to your courtship.
- Be honest yet fair. Yes, honesty hurts, but how else do we change in marriage?
- Don't make assumptions. Check them out. Respond only to what is spoken, not what you're assuming.
- Don't have an "I'm right and you're wrong" attitude about the argument. Realize that each of you may perceive or recall an event very differently. Agree to disagree if necessary. Try to compromise or meet each other half way.

References

Fair fighting rules. Humane Medicine 9:331, 1993

McKay M, Davis M, Fanning P: Messages: The Communication Skill Book. Oakland, CA, New Harbinger Press, 1983

Myers MF: Doctors' Marriages: A Look at the Problems and Their Solutions, 2nd Edition. New York, Plenum, 1994, pp 50–51

Sager CJ: Marriage Contracts and Couple Therapy. New York, Brunner/ Mazel, 1976, pp 19–20

Tannen D: You Just Don't Understand: Women and Men in Conversation. New York, Ballantine, 1990

TWO
Marriage and
the Life Cycle

Critical stages in the individual life cycle closely relate to critical stages in marriage. These stages are normal points of unrest or struggle common to most people in marriage. Therefore, we need to consider the stage of life and/or the stage of marriage of a couple to understand their marital conflict. We should not merely implicate ourselves or our spouses (i.e., individual psychopathology) or the relationship (i.e., marital pathology) and conclude that the marriage is over when it may not be. Individual and marital life cycles are divided into the following seven stages.

Stages of Life Cycles

Stage 1 (early 20s)

The individual stage involves pulling up roots from home and developing autonomy and independence from one's family of origin. If a marital relationship exists, the task is to shift one's allegiance and connectedness from the family to one's spouse, thereby forging a new commitment. This takes time because while one is separating from the family of origin, he or she is simultaneously adjusting to marriage. There may be a number of conflicts with one's parents at this stage as well as with one's in-laws.

Stage 2 (late 20s)

The individual stage is provisional adulthood and the challenge is to identify with one's job or career while developing an increasing capacity for intimacy. Commitment to marriage also can feel provisional, with periods of uncertainty about one's choice of marital partner. There may be corresponding stress with adjustment to parenthood. Work and family may be in opposition for both men and women.

Stage 3 (turning 30)

The individual stage as one makes the age 30 transition involves making a decision about a commitment to one's work and one's marriage. There may be feelings of restlessness and doubt about remaining in the marriage, especially if the partners' paths seem to be diverging. Marital intimacy may suffer with increasing distance; one or both partners may have an extramarital affair.

Stage 4 (30s)

This is a settling-down stage of individual development. It means that there is an increasing ability to deepen one's commitments and to pursue long-range goals. The marital stage is one of productivity—bearing and rearing children, working with vigor, making good friends, and consolidating one's marriage. There may be conflict between the marital partners' ways of achieving productivity. In "good" marriages, there is a marked increase in intimacy; in "bad" marriages, there is gradual distancing.

Stage 5 (early 40s)

This is the beginning of the individual stage of midlife transition. The challenge is searching for the "fit" between one's aspirations and the reality of one's environment. The marital task is one of summing up: success and failure are evaluated and future goals are sought. Husbands and wives may perceive success differently. Indeed, there may be a conflict between one's individual pursuit of success and remaining in one's marriage. Intimacy may be variable.

Stage 6 (mid-40s until mid-60s)

The individual stage is middle adulthood and this includes a restabilizing and reordering of one's priorities. The marital task is to resolve conflicts and to stabilize the marriage for the long haul. There may be differences between husbands and wives in their rates and directions of emotional growth. There may be problems with the loss of youthfulness, resulting in depression or in initiating affairs. Intimacy may be threatened by the aging process and by boredom in the marriage, despite stability and security. Children leaving the parental home may increase or decrease intimacy.

Stage 7 (mid-60s and above)

The individual stage is aging. The individual task at this age is dealing effectively with aging, illness, and death while retaining a zest for life. The marital task is to support each other and to facilitate each other's struggle to be productive and fulfilled in the face of aging. Marital conflict may arise because of rekindled fears of desertion, loneliness, and sexual failure. Many family members and friends die at this stage of the marriage.

Any attempt to describe complicated life events can suffer from being too schematic or simplistic. These seven stages describe people who marry in their early 20s; the current average age at marriage has risen, with many people not marrying until their 30s.

What Has Changed?

Individual stages and tasks within a marriage are no longer as gender free as once thought; we now know much more about unique developmental issues for men and for women. The economic structure of marriage (most marriages currently are dual earner, some also dual career) has changed tremendously. Therefore, marital tasks for women and men are highly influenced by the balance of paid work outside the home and time with family. Men and women are not marrying as young as they once did and they (especially men) are marrying a second or third time more commonly now than 20 years ago. Therefore, some of the marital tasks will be executed at a later stage of the individual life cycle.

Another way of looking at the blending of the individual life cycle and the marital life cycle is to ask the question "Why do people marry?" Once individuals attain a stable identity, it was thought, they marry out of a need and capacity for intimacy with another person. Marriage is a commitment people make to one another and a sharing of parts of themselves. However, in the real world, how many people have really attained "a stable identity" when they get married? How many people are really capable of mature "intimacy" at marriage? This is where one's life stage at the time of marriage becomes quite important. A common statement I hear from individuals who are older and now in a second or third marriage is "I was so young when I got married the first time. I really didn't know myself. I wasn't old enough to fully understand the responsibilities of being a husband (or wife), of being a parent, of really loving in a mature way. This marriage is so different."

There are also gender differences between men and women in the reasons they marry. Women more often define themselves in terms of their relationships, which helps to explain most women's concern with connection and communication in their marriages and their more frequent requests for marital help based on these concerns. Men also desire connection, but they fear it. As part of normal male development boys learn that healthy growth occurs outside of relationships, outside of connection. There is much emphasis on strength, self-sufficiency, achievement, and independence. When men marry, they usually feel more competent at work than at communicating with their wives.

Many people marry for security—financial, physical, and psychological. Some people are really saying, "I don't feel complete without a partner or spouse." Young people fleeing from unhappy homes, in which they may have felt unloved or have been abused, enter marriage with the hope for completion: "I will feel secure and fulfilled with a husband (or wife)." Unfortunately, if the individuals marrying are young or if they are insecure, marriage will not likely provide an enduring solution to their unhappiness and anxiety. That has to come from within, and it takes time.

Most people also marry to have children. This corresponds with a stage called generativity. Again, this is an example of when one's stage of life and one's stage of marriage intersect. One member of the couple may feel that these two are in synchrony but his or her spouse doesn't. They may even be the same,

She Says . . .

"My husband's not very affectionate. The only time he touches me is when he wants sex, and that's become a turnoff. There's no tenderness or sensitivity to my pleasure. Sometimes it even hurts."

This is an extremely common complaint and one filled with misunderstanding. Variants of this complaint are "A hug always turns into a grope." Or, "I'm not a prude, I love oral sex, but not at the front door or in the kitchen, especially with a 2-year-old screaming for attention." Or, "My husband has this habit of coming up behind me when I'm cooking or working at the sink and cupping his hands over my breasts. I hate it and usually swear at him. He thinks I'm frigid."

All of these have a theme—they are unwanted sexual overtures. Yet most men do not see this as their problem; they see it as their wife's problem. They think they are being affectionate, but it is a form of erotic affection that is not consensual and not appropriate for the context. Women develop a learned response of repulsion, which causes them to physically reject their husbands or avoid being near them. This, in turn, makes their husbands feel insecure, unloved, and pushed away.

or nearly the same, biological age, yet one of them may be ready for children and the other not. This is especially applicable to women who feel "the biological clock ticking" but whose husbands do not experience any degree of urgency. Or this could be a marriage in which one is older and ready for procreation but the other is several years younger. Or the other way around—the older person already has one family by an earlier marriage but is ambivalent about a second family with his or her younger (and possibly childless) new spouse.

People also marry for social reasons; that is, they succumb, in part, to the pressures of their families to get married or to societal prescriptions and rules that "being married is normal, being single is not." As ridiculous or outdated as these ideas sound, they aren't so silly when people who aren't married begin to tell their personal stories of how stigmatized they feel. This group includes a range of individuals—the never married, the divorced, many gay and lesbian individuals, and the widowed. Again, life-cycle phases are important here; it is fine to be single until a certain age but not fine after this arbitrary age and stage of life.

Questions About Life/Marital Stages

The following are common questions and statements of married people that touch on life-stage and marital-stage issues.

"I'm 32, my wife is 30; we've been married for 10 years and we have two daughters, 10 and 8. I'm not sure I want to be married anymore. Is this a stage I'm going through?"

Good question! You are trying to understand why you feel uncertain about remaining married. You may feel surprised that you are uncertain. You may be wondering if this is a common feeling in men your age who have been married 10 years. You may also be looking for reassurance that what you are feeling is "normal" or "common" and that it will pass, that within a few months or more, you'll be feeling back on track, in love with your wife, committed, reasonably happy, and so on.

I have several questions for you. These will help me (and you) to explore what is happening. What do you mean by "I'm not sure I want to be married anymore?" There must be reasons why you feel this way. Are you tired of the responsibility? Does being on your own as a single man have some appeal to you—living alone (perhaps for the first time in your life), not having to answer to anyone, peace and quiet more of the time, freedom to date new women, etc.? Are you unhappy with your wife? Bored? Or bitter and angry? Is there enough fun, shared interest, companionship in your marriage? Do you have enough independence and alone time in your marriage? How's your sexual relationship with your wife? Is your lovemaking too infrequent for you or not pleasurable?

Are you depressed and do you find yourself uncertain about a lot of things? For example, are you also fed up with your job and want or need a change? Do you like where you are living or have a wish to be living somewhere else? Are you bored with your friends? Do you feel like you're in a rut? Are you especially critical these days and finding fault with lots of things, including yourself? If the answer to several of these questions is "yes," then don't make a decision about your marriage in isolation. Talk to someone to get another perspective on your mood, because if you are depressed you will be viewing many aspects of your life through dark glasses. Marriage is too big a part of one's life to make a hasty decision.

You married quite young. Could it be that you feel you missed a lot of your youth or that you didn't have enough time to really "sow your oats"? To just have lots of fun and not be so grown up? Do you feel you did enough dating or had enough sexual experience before getting married? Is that something that you envy when you see other men who are dating?

You also mention that you have two children, so you quickly had to give up being single and come to grips with being a husband and a father. That's not easy and something with which most men would struggle. You and your wife had to learn your new roles simultaneously—being husband and wife and father and mother—rather than in tandem. As much as you love your kids, you may regret not having a few years together as a childless couple before starting a family. It's normal to feel that way and it helps just to be able to say it. Life doesn't go as orderly for all of us as we wish it would.

Suggestions

So back to your question: Is this a stage I'm going through? Maybe . . . or maybe not. At the age 30 transition it's common to question one's life and very common to do so after 7 or more years of marriage. What's important is that you talk about it. Talk to your wife about it. She may feel the same way. Remember she was only 20 when she got married! My hunch is that she may have many feelings similar to yours. She may not be considering separation, but she may have some suggestions for how to deal with these feelings. My hope is that a dialogue between the two of you might help clarify things and also promote more closeness and understanding, especially if you or each of you has been feeling distant, unloved, unappreciated, dismissed, rejected, bored, or angry with things.

Also talk with someone other than your wife: a close friend, a sibling, your mother or father, a mentor, a colleague at work. Be sure this is someone you respect for his or her listening ability, acceptance, trustworthiness, maturity, and wisdom. Just opening up to someone about this may help tremendously. The feelings may pass, allowing you to move to a deeper level of acceptance of your life.

If things seem more difficult than this, and you feel a pervasive sense of unhappiness at home or you feel depressed and despairing, you're beginning to drink excessively, you're avoiding family life, or you're having an affair, I suggest that you turn to professional help. You need someone with objectivity, training, and experience to help you understand what's happening. This same person can also be your guide as you explore options and solutions.

"**W**e're not very happy together. We bicker a lot these days, and our lives are more and more separate. I'm 50; Bob is 51. Since his affair last year, I don't trust him anymore. We've been married 25 years."

So what's going on here? Were your lives diverging before your husband's affair, or has it happened since the affair, or both? If your lives were fairly separate before Bob met the other woman, then that might have contributed to his beginning the affair. He was vulnerable, lonely, empty, bored, or restless. Perhaps he had even given some thought to separation but abandoned the idea with the resolve to just "hang in." If your marriage actually seemed reasonably close and fairly vital before your husband's affair, and if he shares that perception, then the reasons for his affair may be quite different. (I'll return to this in a moment.) If your lives have only felt separate *since* Bob's affair, then there are unresolved issues associated with it. These need to be addressed, probably with marital therapy. If your separateness feels like a bit of both, that is, some separateness before the affair and some since, then a number of interacting factors need uncovering and resolution if you are to feel happy and confident again about your relationship.

Your bickering and unhappiness are probably connected to this sense of separateness. It may even feel like a vicious cycle to you. That is, the more you poke and snipe at each other, the more you avoid each other (because it's so unpleasant). However, the more you avoid being together, the less opportunity you have for comfortable peaceful time together, which can offset the bad times and restore hopefulness. Therefore, the bulk of the time you have together is negative. And who wants that?

The fact that you don't trust your husband is not surprising. Whenever one's basic trust in marriage has been shattered by an outside relationship, it always takes a lot of dialogue, disclosure of information, uncovering of possible reasons for the affair, explanation for any lying and/or deceit, release of anger and hurt, expression of remorse and guilt, reassurance that one is indeed loved, and passage of time (for most people, at least a year) before it feels that trust is returning. And even then, trust can be quite ephemeral. It can be temporarily derailed if there is any incident where the facts don't quite jibe, or one is late or unavailable when he or she should be. When it is possible to restore trust, it takes time and hard work.

I wonder how much talking you and your husband have done about his affair; whether you have the assurance that it is truly over, whether you feel confident that your husband wants to be with you, and whether your level of communication, affection, and sexuality together are good. Do you really understand why it happened and feel quite confident that it won't happen again? Some spouses can state this with marked certainty and sincerity, whereas others cannot. Second extramarital affairs in marriage are very uncommon when or if the first one has resulted in a marital crisis and both parties have worked hard at dealing with it and forging a new level of trust, communication, and deep intimacy.

Now, let's look at the perception that you and your husband considered your marriage quite good, and yet he had the affair. Perhaps he was having a so-called midlife crisis in which he felt uncertain about many things in his life—his job, his marriage, his family, and so forth. This inner turmoil, coupled with a fear of aging, can set the stage for an affair—an affair that makes it all go away, that makes the person feel happy, revitalized, younger, more energetic, forward thinking, creative, and interesting. The pull can seem magnetic and overpowering. One's personal judgment and previously conservative value system can fly out the window.

Another possibility is the presence of a psychiatric illness that renders a spouse more susceptible to having an affair. Examples are depression, bipolar illness (manic-depression), alcoholism and drug abuse, and organic brain disease (like dementia, which affects a person's reasoning, memory, or judgment). In other words, the person wouldn't normally get involved with someone else were he or she feeling well, but because of a psychiatric illness, he or she is more vulnerable to the attraction of someone else, the temptations that most people normally resist. The person's neediness is greater than usual for time, attention, support, love, or sex. He or she is not functioning with the usual level of energy, purpose, self-control, conscience, reservation, and caution.

None of the above is intended as an excuse. My goal in explaining an affair from a psychiatric perspective is not to make excuses for the behavior. It simply recasts "bad" behavior into "symptomatic" behavior. Rage is a normal reaction. You can still be angry at a spouse who had an affair, even if he or she was psychiatrically ill at the time!

Suggestions

As both you and your husband consider the above, note if there is some resonance to your personal situation, then formulate some questions to ask each other. Approach him and say that the two of you need to talk, that you are not comfortable with your feelings about the marriage, that, despite your best intentions, you do not trust him very much. This may hurt him or make him angry, but those emotions are all part of communication about such a serious matter. Do not let him stonewall you into silence. If you feel that happening, say so. Also tell him that if you are not allowed to talk about your feelings about his affair, you cannot see any way out of this state of mistrust and distance.

Give some thought to marital therapy. A couples therapist is trained to assist the two of you in discussing painful subjects, like extramarital relationships. Bring this up with your husband. If he demurs, his main reason will probably be the dread of "dredging up the past." Tell him that you understand but that perhaps it would be a bit easier with a guide who can keep the dialogue on track and the emotion within acceptable boundaries. The therapist should also be able to assist the two of you in uncovering the reasons for the affair.

You might also consider psychotherapy for yourself alone, especially if your husband refuses to accompany you to marital therapy and nothing is working. This will provide you with some perspective on your marriage, its health, your role in the marriage, and what you are deriving from it. You may also feel a sense of support as you evolve through this period. If you have been blaming yourself, your self-esteem should improve as well, along with your assertiveness, if that has been a problem for you.

Your husband, too, might give some thought to psychotherapy with the goal of understanding himself better. Its focus could be his affair, but there are likely other conflicts and issues that are a struggle for him. A positive experience with a therapist should also help him speak to you with more clarity, honesty, and vitality.

"I'm 63 and I wish my husband would retire. My arthritis is getting worse and worse each year. I would like to do some traveling while I still can. My husband and I argue a lot about money and about our kids—they've all had a lot of problems the past couple of years."

You sound unhappy and understandably weary. You have reached a stage in your life and marriage when you expected to have more time with your husband for companionship. Yet he's still working, probably pretty hard. Your arthritis is worsening and threatening your ability to travel with some measure of independence and flexibility. If the stress of your marriage (arguing about money) and the worry about your kids are making your arthritis worse, this is all the more reason to have relaxation time with your husband.

If your husband plans to retire soon, a lot of your worry will be eliminated. But if he has no intention of retiring or keeps putting it off, this needs to be addressed. What does work mean to him? How much of his self-worth and purpose emanate from his work? How much is financial? You mentioned that the two of you argue about money. Is he worried about savings and whether there's enough for retirement? Are your dreams of travel shared by him or does he think travel is too expensive?

You also mention that the two of you argue a lot about your kids. Are your arguments rooted in worry about them? Are you blaming yourselves or each other for their problems? Don't forget that your children are adults and are responsible for their own lives. You can love them and support them, but their problems are not your fault. You mentioned kids and money in the same sentence. Are your kids dependent on you and your husband financially? If so, this pressure may be a factor in your husband's continuing to work and not taking retirement.

Suggestions

Try to approach your husband in a manner least likely to make him defensive. Explaining your worsening arthritis to him is a good place to start. He needs to know how limited you're beginning to feel in terms of your physical mobility, how much pain and stiffness you have, how demoralized you get at times, and how much you feel a sense of time urgency. If you feel he will not or cannot hear you on this, take him with you to your next medical appointment. Your husband might be more responsive to getting the message from your doctor concerning what the future holds. If the picture is not as grim as you believe, you will feel relieved and so will your husband. And he may still be interested in traveling.

See if you and your husband can reach a middle ground on when and how he retires. Are there any other options? Can he semiretire? Can he retire from his field but still keep active with secondary work, volunteer work, or personal pursuits? If a large part of your husband's identity is related to his work, it may be more palatable for him to give it up gradually.

Don't back away from your wish to have more time with your husband. Don't let him use work as an excuse. Many men who work full-time into their 60s and 70s cut back from *overwork* and enjoy relaxation time with their wives. This is the stage of life to be doing activities together. What you long for and expect are normal.

"Is it normal to feel disillusioned after being married a few years?"

Absolutely. Part of being human is buying into the mythology that our spouses are going to be perfect and meet all of our needs, that we will feel whole, happy, and at relative peace. This is a carryover from childhood, when we expected our parents to meet those needs and then felt angry when they didn't. To find that marriage can be very stressful, confusing, and at times so full of conflict can be upsetting and very disappointing. We wonder: Did I make a mistake? Did I marry the wrong person? Should I have gotten married at all? Is there someone else out there who will love me more, who will find me more attractive, more sexually desirable, who will be a better listener, who will accept my flaws, who will be stronger, who will be more ambitious, or who doesn't smoke?

It is normal for these feelings of disillusionment to come and go, on and off, during the early years of marriage. They are especially common during a tense or difficult time together or accompanying or following an argument. But if they pass relatively quickly, especially after a good talk, then there is nothing to worry about. It is when feelings of disillusionment persist for weeks, months, or years that they are a sign of something amiss that needs attention. They should be talked about with your spouse, with a close and trusted family member or friend, or with a professional such as your family doctor, a member of the clergy, or a psychotherapist.

These feelings could mean many things. They could mean that you are in a life or marital stage that is temporary and normal, or that you or your spouse are under a lot of stress and it is affecting your marriage, or that you are depressed. They could indicate that your marriage is in trouble and needs marital therapy, or that your marriage is over, that it is no longer working, or that it never really worked in the first place and you and your spouse are incompatible.

"What's a biological clock? Do both women and men have it?"

The term *biological clock* is used to refer to the consciousness that women possess toward their reproductive capacity. When a woman says "My biological clock is running out," what she is saying is, "I don't have much time left to have a child before my chances of conceiving are greatly reduced." Women begin to pay heed to their biological clocks in their mid to late 30s and certainly by their 40s. Quite understandably, a woman's decision to have a child, or another child, must be crystallized by this period.

Men do not have a biological clock. They can inseminate a woman well into late life, perhaps not so readily, but fertilization is certainly possible. What men do have though is a *psychological* clock. They reach a stage of life when they want to have a child and a later stage when they don't. Some men never have a period in their life when they want children. This can be the same for women.

Conflict arises when there is a difference in the "clocks." He is ready to start a family and she isn't. Or she is ready to conceive and he isn't. She may be ready in part because of her biological clock— she feels that time is running out. He doesn't have to worry about a biological clock, so he can afford to wait until he is psychologically ready. This can be extremely frustrating for both parties. She is frustrated because he is negative or resistant to having a child now and seemingly unsympathetic to her sense of urgency. He may argue that she is too worried about her biological clock and that there is still lots of time. He gets frustrated because he feels pressured by her to agree to having a child before he is psychologically or perhaps financially ready.

Conflict around this matter can become more complicated when the man already has children by a previous marriage and is now in a relationship with someone who has never had children. Hence, her sense of primacy for becoming pregnant may be much greater than his. If he keeps putting her off, she may begin to wonder if he wants more children at all. She may feel duped and resentful, emotions that upset him and perhaps alienate him from her.

What I want to emphasize here is the normality of this stage of life and marriage. Whether it's a biological or a psychological clock that individuals are observing, their clocks may not be synchronized. The solution is to keep talking about it, over and over, until some compromise is reached. Both parties must be willing to give somewhat. If this seems impossible, therapy may help to break the impasse and to restore relationship morale and confidence. In some situations, the only solution is separation.

"My wife is depressed. Could it be the menopause?"

It may be a contributor, but menopause alone does not give women a distinct or inevitable depression. Indeed, menopause may be a facilitator of excellent mental health for many women. The combination of hormonal and psychological factors correspond with other changes in a woman's life, for example, her children growing up and leaving home. It is a time of renewal when women who have put many of their personal needs and wishes on hold for their husbands and children are freed up to pursue their desires.

On the other hand, for a few women menopause is truly experienced as a loss—a loss of fertility, of course, and a loss of youthful beauty and attractiveness. This can occur in happily married women whose husbands are naturally complimentary and sensitive. It is in part a by-product of the youth-oriented society in which we live (aging is bad) and the common fact that many men in their middle years are attracted to younger women. "It's pretty demoralizing to be at a 'singles' event and to observe most of the men your age talking to women 10 years younger," said a divorced 49-year-old woman. We are products of the culture in which we live. It is a struggle to constantly fight "menopausal myths," which may eventually erode self-esteem.

Your wife, however, may be depressed for other reasons that have nothing to do with menopause. Ask her what she thinks about it. How much might be biological? Has she had depression before? Is there a family history? Is her drinking a problem? Is she taking any medication that could be making her feel depressed? How is her general medical health? How's your marriage—is she worried about the two of you? How are your children? Are there money worries? If she's working outside the home, are there any problems at work? Discussing all of these subjects might be helpful; you both may end up feeling better. If your wife agrees with your perception of depression, she should visit her physician.

"What's the empty nest syndrome?"

Empty nest syndrome refers to the change of family composition in the home when the children grow up and leave. Now the family at home is comprised of only two adults—the original two people who met, married, and produced a family. When people think of the empty nest syndrome, they usually imagine sadness, loneliness, wistfulness, quiet, boredom, restlessness, and an irrational clinging to the adult children. Marital tension may arise at this time because of the newness of this smaller family.

Originally it was thought that women suffered from empty nest symptoms because their role as full-time mothers had come to an end and they were now at loose ends. However, with more and more women working outside the home while raising their children, there are fewer women who complain of empty nest problems. This, coupled with so many offerings for women (returning to college, doing volunteer work, traveling, returning to paid work), gives women many more opportunities now than a generation ago.

It was also thought that only women developed empty nest symptoms. That simply isn't true. Nowadays more and more men complain of empty nest loneliness and sadness. Men may especially feel this when their wives are very busy with their own personal pursuits and don't have a lot of time for them. It is crucial that men in situations like this begin to make more of a life for themselves by taking up interests of their own or with their friends.

Some men haven't been happy in their marriage for a while and have had many of their needs met by their children (needs for intellectual stimulation, affirmation, companionship, conversation, physical activity). These men experience many empty nest symptoms and, in fact, may have a marital crisis at this stage of life and find themselves very unhappy at home. They hadn't realized this earlier because they were so caught up in their children's lives and hadn't paid too much attention to their marriage. Arguments, fights, distancing, an affair—these are all possibilities at this time. Marital therapy can be very helpful in delineating the issues and seeing what can be done about them. If successful adjustment to this stage of marriage does not occur, separation and divorce may be the only options for regaining one's mental health.

"My wife and I don't have sex anymore. We've been married 30 years. Is that abnormal?"

As a psychiatrist, I have a problem with the word *abnormal.* So please allow me to change the word to *uncommon.* No, it's not uncommon to no longer have sex after 30 years of marriage. It doesn't matter if you are 50 or 70 years old; age is not the issue. Perhaps you wonder if you and your wife are OK, and not neurotic, or sick, or in denial about the importance of sex in an enduring relationship. You may also be asking, "Should we be worried about us, about our future together, about our individual sexual needs, about the risk of an affair for one or both of us?" Very likely, the answer is "No, you've got nothing to worry about."

That said, let me explore two possibilities with you: 1) you are quite happily married and both of you are fine about no longer being sexual together; 2) one of you is not happy about the lack of sex in your relationship. This partner has asked the question because he or she is at war about this and wants to find out who is right, who is wrong, who is normal, who is "abnormal."

In the first instance, you and your wife have come to a stated or unstated agreement to stop having sex. I do not know what your sexual life was like through the course of your marriage. Perhaps it was very good and mutually satisfying but sex no longer interests either of you or feels necessary. Those years of sexual intimacy are now behind you and offer you pleasant memories. On the other hand, your sexual life together could have been strained and troubling for the two of you, so to be no longer sexual may be a bit of a relief; something that caused tension, arguments, or sadness no longer interrupts your marital equilibrium. You can show your love for each other in many ways outside of the bedroom. And if you are both satisfied by this, and not lonely or resentful, I doubt if either of you is at risk for an extramarital affair.

In the second situation, in which one of you is not happy about the sexual relationship ending, I would be concerned. It is not good enough to simply leave it like this or to solicit the opinion of an expert who may or may not agree with one of you. Experts' comments probably run the gamut from "It's OK not to have sex after 30 years of marriage" to "It's never OK."

You need to keep talking about this. What is going on? Try to see if you can come to some compromise. For example, is there a nonsexual way of expressing your love and affection for each other? A way that still involves some physical touch and closeness? Holding hands can feel very reassuring to someone who has felt rejected and unloved in a marriage that no longer has a sexual connection. Going for walks and taking your partner's arm can also be reassuring. A light kiss and a warm embrace at the beginning and the end of each day can be soothing. If these physical gestures don't help, consider talking to a therapist together. He or she may have some ideas that will help.

"Don't you think it's cruel to get divorced after 40 years of marriage?"

Not necessarily. Surprising and sad, yes. But cruel? It depends a lot on the specifics. If one of the partners has especially wanted the separation and divorce, and the other is dead against it and feels devastated and abandoned, yes, it can appear cruel to that person and his or her friends and family. But what must not be overlooked in this couple's separation are their personal and marital dynamics. It is quite possible, if not probable, that the one who is leaving has been miserable for a long time. Divorce at this stage of life may be liberating and may offer the person the potential for peace and/or inner happiness for the remaining years of life.

The word *cruel* implies blame and judgment. In other words, the person leaving is charged with doing a very bad thing to the spouse. To want to leave a 40-year marriage implies selfishness and no remorse about inflicting hurt and pain on one's partner. Most separations at this stage of life are not like this—there is remorse, reflection, and caring for the person left behind. Unless one takes the time to listen to the stories of both parties, who really knows the specifics of the marriage and the separation?

When observers accuse the person who is leaving of being cruel, there may be circumstances that point in that direction. Perhaps the one leaving left abruptly with no clear warning to his or her spouse. Perhaps the spouse is physically or mentally disabled (anyone who has lived in a marriage like this can attest to the hardship and demoralization that may be present). Perhaps the one leaving has not been fair about financial support. Perhaps there is a third party, and, if so, maybe this affair hasn't been conducted discretely, that is, the extramarital relationship has been "flaunted," causing humiliation to the spouse.

So there may be elements of cruelty in some cases. Perhaps the divorce might have been handled in a better or more sensitive way. Yet a person who is "left" may take up a victim role in response to many life stressors, so that no matter how graciously the spouse tries to leave, he or she is going to be portrayed as a mean and thoughtless person.

"Why do so many men marry younger women the second time around?"

This is a complex question with no single or easy answer. Some men admit that they love the recognition, or envious glances, they get from their male friends and colleagues at work, that it is like being a teenager and walking tall "because they've got the best-looking girl." Some men respond that they deliberately sought out a younger woman because they like the physical beauty of younger people, or the energy, or the freshness, or the adoring affection and naiveté of someone younger. There is also the potential for a second family and more children. Or it may be the sex—sex that is more frequent, exciting, uninhibited, and more fulfilling.

These are all surface responses. Some men will say that their being with someone younger is purely accidental or serendipitous, that they just met and fell in love with each other, and that they were not deliberately looking for someone younger than themselves. This is especially common when men meet women in the workplace or in social settings like gyms, singles' bars and clubs, and so on. Very often, women their own age are home with children, and their former husbands are in the same settings as other men—around younger, single women.

Another factor is that some women are drawn to older men whom they meet through work or in social venues. The attraction is to someone who seems more mature, who is settled into a career, who is earning good money, who seems more sensitive to their needs, who is a more experienced lover, who seems like a good father (when or if he has kids). The reservation rests in the complicated dynamics of getting involved with someone who has so many other responsibilities that take his time, energy, and money—time that is not available to the woman.

At a deeper level, marrying a younger woman enables some men to deny their own aging process. "I feel young again and I have a new lease on life." "I thought my life was over—I'm born again, without all the religion." "Our sex life is a gift; I feel like a 20-year-old stud." "I love being a father again, especially now that I have the time to be a father—I was working so hard when I had kids in my first marriage that I missed their childhood." "I hope my health remains good; I really don't want to become a burden on my wife or not to be able to ski and play tennis with my kids." These are some statements from male patients of mine who are married to younger women.

"My new girlfriend wants kids of her own. Should I get my vasectomy reversed?"

This is a common dilemma for many men; men who thought they were finished having children when they had the procedure originally done or men who thought that their marriage was secure and stable. Even if they saw some problems and the possibility of divorce, these men never thought they would consider having more children. Being in love and in a new relationship can change all of that.

My suggestion is that the two of you take considerable time to think about this decision. It is very serious. You need to rethink your life plan. Do more kids, and the attendant responsibility, appeal to you? You need to be very honest with yourself about this, and if the answer is no, the relationship must end unless she can forego her original life plan and accept being a stepmother to your children and not have her own.

In this chapter I have tried to illustrate that we have cycles and stages in our lives that color our thoughts, feelings, hopes, and dreams regarding our love relationships. What preoccupies us and what we decide at one stage of life may be very different than what we do at another stage. It is easier to see our way clear when we understand that a lot of our confusion is common, normal, and time limited.

References

Berman EM, Lief HI: Marital therapy from a psychiatric perspective: an overview. American Journal of Psychiatry 132:583–592, 1975

Erikson EH: Childhood and Society, 2nd Edition. New York, WW Norton, 1963

Gilligan C: In a Different Voice: Psychological Theory and Women's Development. Cambridge, MA, Harvard University Press, 1982

Myers MF: Men and Divorce. New York, Guilford, 1989

Myers MF: Men's unique developmental issues across the life cycle, in American Psychiatric Press Review of Psychiatry, Vol 10. Edited by Tasman A, Goldfinger SM. Washington, DC, American Psychiatric Press, 1991, pp 578–593

Notman MT, Klein R, Jordan JV, et al: Women's unique developmental issues across the life cycle, in American Psychiatric Press Review of Psychiatry, Vol 10. Edited by Tasman A, Goldfinger SM. Washington, DC, American Psychiatric Press, 1991, pp 556–577

THREE

Sexual Problems

Our sex life just isn't what it was" is one of the most common complaints couples bring to marital therapists. But what does this mean?

Some couples have noticed a change in how frequently they make love. They are concerned that what they believe to be a major aspect of being married is losing its position of importance in their lives together. Often the change in frequency of lovemaking is viewed as a problem by only one partner. For example, he may worry or get angry or depressed about it but she doesn't feel there has been that much of a change, or, if she does, she may dismiss it as nothing serious or even as a relief in some way. This different way of experiencing a changed lovemaking frequency may in itself upset marital equilibrium. The couple may conclude that this is just another example of where they no longer see eye to eye—or where one feels dismissed by the other.

Another meaning attached to changes in one's sex life is that sex has become routine or boring. "We always use the missionary position. I'd like to experiment a bit but my husband doesn't want to." What this woman is actually saying is that what used to be very exciting isn't any longer. If both agree that sex has become routine, it is easier to make changes. But it is harder if one partner is quite satisfied or if one does not make changes easily.

Some couples complain that the sex they share is great, but it's not very loving or intimate. One man said, "We've probably got the hottest sex on our block—neither of us is uptight or shy—we've tried every position, oral sex, anal sex, dildos, porn movies, S & M, you name it, we've done it—but there seems to be something missing despite orgasms that are a 7 on the Richter scale and have each of us screaming for more!" This illustrates that sex and intimacy do not always go hand in hand, that it is possible to be sexually satisfied but not feel close or intimate with your partner. Some couples even say, "All we've got going for us is great sex—the rest of our relationship sucks." Also, some couples who are separating, are separated, or are divorcing describe great sex that is uncontaminated by their relationship that is unraveling and disengaging in every other way.

Another meaning of the complaint that "our sex life just isn't what it was" is that sex is no longer arousing or it is just barely arousing. He might complain that it takes him a long time to get an erection or when he does, he loses it easily. Or perhaps he gets erections easily enough but it's hard for him to ejaculate; that is, despite a lot of stimulation, it takes him a long time to come or maybe he can't come

---

He Says, She Says . . .

He says: "My wife complains that I'm a terrible communicator. She always wants to know my feelings."

She says: "My husband's one of those quiet types. I don't know what he's thinking half the time or if he's upset about something."

Many wives today are frustrated with the way their husbands talk to them (or don't talk to them). They state that they are always having to read between the lines, or second-guess, or pull information, or force it. Some men argue that we are living in an era when "expressing feeling" is thought to be the only way or the best way to communicate and for men to adopt a "female" way of communicating may not always be possible or even appropriate.

Why is it so difficult for men to disclose feelings? The question is complex and has biological, psychological, and cultural underpinnings. More specifically, men feel vulnerable when, or if, they express their feelings about a marital concern. And when they feel vulnerable, they usually feel frightened that they're losing control, inviting attack, criticism, humiliation, or abandonment. Some men, in fact, will argue that they've never shared their feelings with anyone and ask their wives not to take it personally.

at all with intercourse. She, on the other hand, may say that she rarely has orgasms anymore, and when she does they're not like they used to be—they are brief, single rather than multiple, less intense, physical, and not very emotional. Or she may not be orgasmic at all and not understand why that is, especially if she is having orgasms easily when masturbating.

Some couples have begun to experience their sex life together as physically painful. He may complain of pain in his penis after intercourse or pain in his testicles or prostate area. She may have vaginal pain during or after intercourse. Or she may experience vaginal constriction at the beginning of intercourse so that her husband may not be able to enter her—or if he does, it hurts her, especially when he makes thrusting movements. This feels paradoxical to some couples, who say, "I think we're going backwards. Aren't couples more likely to have these kinds of sexual problems when they're young and uptight about sex? We're in our 40s and have kids. Shouldn't we be over this stuff now?" Not necessarily. Unpleasant emotions in marriage as well as individual medical problems can contribute to sexual pain and discomfort in certain people.

Finally, this is a subject that is not easy for most couples to talk about. It is very personal. To conclude that "our sex life just isn't what it was" can cause people to feel guilty, blamed, and very defensive. Even if one partner isn't actually blaming the other, he or she may *feel* blamed or accused of being inadequate, uninterested, or unloving. This misunderstanding can lead to fighting, crying, recriminations, and withdrawal, which may dampen what was present in a positive sense—their caring, loving, and mutual respect for each other.

What Is a Sexual Dysfunction?

This rather awkward, clinical term refers to individuals with one or more of three sexual concerns: problems of desire or interest in sex, problems of arousal (lubrication troubles in women and erection troubles in men), and problems of orgasm or climax (inability to experience orgasm in women and premature ejaculation or retarded ejaculation in men). I will not go into detail about these three concerns except to mention that couples with marital problems can have any of these types of sexual problems. But by far the most common in couples whose marriage is distressed are disorders of sexual desire. This makes sense, because who feels like making love if you're really angry, or hurt, or not trusting of your spouse?

Because sexual dysfunction tends to be complicated and may have physical and/or psychological causes, let me suggest the following: If you have one of these sexual concerns, go to your physician for a complete medical history and physical examination. He or she will be able to recommend whether you should next see a specialist, a gynecologist or urologist, an endocrinologist, a sexual medicine specialist (usually a physician or nurse), a sex therapist (usually a psychologist), or a marital therapist. I can't emphasize this enough. There are many medical conditions, psychiatric disorders, medications, and stress-related states that can affect how we feel and respond sexually.

Because I am a psychiatrist *and* a marital therapist, most couples who come to me with sexual concerns are having problems related to a medical/psychiatric disorder, relationship difficulties, or both. In other words, sex is usually only one of several concerns and most often seems to be a result of marital tension and unhappiness or depression. One or both do not feel like making love, or if they do, the quality of their sexual loving is not what it used to be. Their unhappiness, tension, hurt, anger, or mistrust of each other has affected their sexual life as a couple.

Sex therapists, on the other hand, primarily see couples who have happy, healthy marriages but who are experiencing sexual difficulties. In other words, these couples communicate reasonably well, love each other, are committed to each other, are not sitting on anger and hurt, trust each other, and are motivated to improve things in the sexual realm of their lives. Here are just some of the reasons behind sexual difficulties:

- Naiveté or lack of information about normal sexual functioning and practice
- Sexual shyness, embarrassment, and rigidity

- Religious or moral constraints against sexual freedom and relaxation within marriage
- Medical disorders such as diabetes, rheumatoid arthritis, multiple sclerosis, thyroid illness, strokes, heart disease, or cancer
- Surgical procedures that can affect one's sexuality, like surgery for cancer of the vulva or vagina or cancer of the prostate
- Traumatic injury to one's spinal cord, like paraplegia or quadriplegia
- Psychological and sexual trauma from having been sexually abused as a child or assaulted as an adult
- Confusion about one's sexual orientation (Am I gay? Am I straight? Am I bisexual?)
- Confusion about one's gender identity (Am I a woman trapped in a man's body? Or vice versa)

Now that I have described some of the more common sexual complaints couples bring to marital therapists, especially complaints that represent a change in the quantity or quality of lovemaking, I want to return to the main theme of this chapter, the relationship between sex and marriage. Let me emphasize again that these complaints must be seen in context—the context of something amiss in the marriage that has created sexual difficulty and concern. This is very important, because to try to "fix" things in the bedroom without understanding why there's a problem in the first place just won't work. The answer is to find out what the causes are and to tackle them. If they can be resolved, very often things improve spontaneously in bed, or sex becomes even better than it used to be.

Common Factors That Affect Sexual Intimacy

Busy Lives

I think this is the most common reason why couples today complain of a change in their sexual relationship. "We just can't seem to find the time to make love" or "When we do, I'm exhausted (or my partner is)." The vast majority of couples in North America are now dual in-come; that is, both are working for pay outside the home. Some cou-ples are both full-time or both part-time or one part-time and one full-time. Some also work different shifts, which means they have fewer hours in the day when they are both home simultaneously and can spend time together. This affects their time in bed, but perhaps more important, they don't have as much time for relaxation or shared leisure, which forms so much of the "foreplay" of sex. Women espe-cially feel less like making love if they've had minimal or no time with their husband before he makes a sexual overture.

However, things are not very different for those couples whose marriages are more traditional—he is the sole wage earner, and she is home full-time as a mother and homemaker. Unpaid work in the home has become as stressful, sometimes more stressful, than paid work. Wives or husbands who are at home full-time spend a lot of time on domestic labor, marketing, driving children from one lesson or event to another, supervising homework and music practice, per-forming the administrative aspects of running the home (i.e., the CEO role in marriage), and doing community and other forms of vol-unteer work. At the end of the day or at the end of the 7-day week, both partners are usually beat, and one or both may just want time alone before bedtime.

Some will argue that all this "busyness" is just an excuse or an es-cape from sexuality in marriage and that men and women are simply running away from each other when it comes to sex. I say "men and women" because even though men complain more than women about the lack of sex or infrequent sex in marriage, they are not pri-oritizing sex, despite their posturing, any higher than women are. Yes, they may feel like having sex more often, they may initiate it more often than their wives, and they may get upset more. But the bottom line is that they are usually just as busy as their wives and they don't make the time to spend "nonsexual" time together.

This argument—that men and women are running away from each other—is largely a cynical position about contemporary mar-riage. In my thinking, it's not fair. True, there are marriages in which sex falters and one or both partners are avoiding sex for conscious or unconscious reasons. This is a case for marital therapy, which will be discussed in more detail in a later chapter. But there are many other couples whose sex life is infrequent because they live highly stressed and fast-paced lives. These couples often say that when they do make love, it's pretty good and they also say that when they take vacations, their sex life together is usually better both in frequency and in satisfaction.

Here are some concluding comments. Most couples state that attempts to "squeeze in" sex at some point in the day or week usually fail. This is understandable because often there just isn't enough time. One of them may be quite preoccupied with matters other than sex and can't relax enough to thoroughly enjoy the sensual experience. The other may feel rushed because of time constraints and feel under pressure to "perform"—and that is no way to enjoy sex. Some couples abhor having to "schedule" sex for the weekends (or days off from work). Yes, there is something terribly unromantic about scheduling sex. However, unless there is communication between two people that perhaps they can do a few things together on the weekend, maybe reconnect and regain some intimacy, and *perhaps* make love, then that day may never come, or may come rarely.

Poor Communication

As the years go on, sexual fulfillment in marriage is increasingly dependent on the ability to talk to each other. If people are too busy to sit down together or to get away together, it is really hard to remain in touch with what is going on in each other's lives, let alone in each other's hearts. The feelings of closeness associated with deep and meaningful communication enhance shared sexuality, as do other results of good communication—a sense of common purpose, commitment to each other, a sense of being supported and comforted, a feeling of safety and protection by and for the other, and an ethos of trust.

When couples don't make the time to sit down and talk, attempts at communication become pressured and time limited, causing misunderstandings and strong negative feelings in both parties. This may cause tension, disagreements, and arguments because there isn't time to thoroughly discuss issues and to reach a compromise or consensus. This makes the idea of communicating unpleasant or tedious because dialogue doesn't flow. The result is that one or both begin to avoid each other. Unfortunately, this only widens the gulf and makes further attempts at communication even more strained. Soon feelings of estrangement ensue in the relationship, both in and out of the bedroom.

Differing Expectations

Another factor that can affect sexual harmony is rooted in a couple's inability to agree on expectations. For example, most couples today say they would rather have less frequent sex as long as it's high quality, that is, enjoyable and pleasurable for both with an enhanced feeling of intimacy. But this won't work if only one of them accepts this or if they can't agree on the frequency of lovemaking. Friction arises if one of them continues to make sexual overtures (which feel like demands) and his or her spouse demurs. If this isn't identified as a problem of communication or honesty of purpose, then tension can affect the good sex life they have been enjoying.

Dishonesty

Dishonest or fraudulent behavior in the bedroom has a very negative effect on intimacy. What I mean by this is role playing by one or both partners. On the surface they seem to have a good sex life and as long as they don't examine it, things may work well, at least for a while. Below the surface, however, there may be a lack of intimacy and distance, hostility, loneliness, and unhappiness. Here are some examples from my practice:

- "I just lie there and let my husband have his fun. Isn't that sort of my job as a wife?"
- "As long as I fantasize about hot women I can get it up."
- "Sometimes I compose my shopping list or just itemize all of the things I have to do the next day."

- "I fake orgasms. I always have."
- "I can't be bothered saying no. It's too much of a hassle. He'll either get angry and he might slap me around a bit or he'll sulk for the next 24 hours. So I just give in. He never takes very long anyway because he's only doing it for his own pleasure, certainly not mine."
- "My wife doesn't know that I'm gay. I'm a master at performing like a stud when we're in bed. She says I'm the best lover she's ever had, and it may be true because satisfying her is very important to me. I can get my own jollies elsewhere."
- "I wonder about our sex life sometimes. What I mean is that the only time we get together is when we've had quite a lot to drink or we're both stoned on marijuana."

The pattern of accommodating to one's spouse seems to be more common in women, but that's understandable. Sexual fakery will continue until women feel safe to be completely honest with their husbands and understand that they have a right to their own sexual likes and dislikes (and their husbands understand this). For some, the consequences of complete honesty are just too dangerous—abandonment, punishment, cheating, shaming, and violence.

Sometimes it's hard to recognize one's true feelings about sex. Something may not feel right, but one can't quite identify what it is: "Why don't I feel as turned on as I used to? Why don't I feel like making love anymore? Why don't I just do it? Lots of things in life require effort; not everything comes easy all of the time."

Some, if not most, married people feel guilty if they don't feel sexually attracted to or satisfied by their spouse. You are supposed to when you're married! In an attempt to deny these feelings in themselves, they find it easier to fantasize or to use drugs that are sexually stimulating to maintain the illusion. Then they don't have to deal with a problem that feels overwhelming but which in reality is very common and one with which most couples struggle at some point in their marriage.

When sex in a marriage becomes fraudulent, life with your partner can become confusing. If you get the sense that your partner is really interested in you physically, it hurts tremendously when things don't seem to be going well elsewhere in the relationship. It just doesn't make sense. Sex can be used as a panacea, a cure-all, a tonic, especially when things are not going smoothly. The unspoken message is "Let's not argue or fight, let's have sex." So problems don't get resolved; they are just glossed over. As one woman said, "Sex is a great escape. My husband and I used it for 5 years. The worse our communication got, the more we had sex, until finally we both realized that our marriage was a sham and always had been. We split up."

Negativity

A negative atmosphere in the home can really get in the way of sex in marriage. By negative I mean a tense, hostile, indifferent, cold, depressing, or bizarre cast that characterizes the relationship. Under these conditions sexual distancing would make sense in light of the interpersonal climate. Fortunately, most couples whose relationship has deteriorated to this point have come to accept that sexual absence or infrequency is inevitable.

There are many reasons why the atmosphere can feel negative at home. Here is one example:

Sara, speaking for both herself and her husband Ted, began their first visit with these words: "We haven't had sex in months. I couldn't care less if we ever made love again. The bottom fell out of our relationship a year ago when Ted lost his job. It's been a downhill mess since. We had a huge mortgage so we had to sell our house and move, which meant I had to close my in-home day care. Our son got kicked out of his new school. He's got attention-deficit hyperactivity disorder and doesn't adapt to change very well. Our daughter got pregnant and had to have an abortion. I've developed migraines, and I'm on all kinds of painkillers. Ted still hasn't found work—and he's drinking more, which I resent, and he knows it. My dad was an abusive alcoholic. We're on welfare—it's humiliating—and we can't make ends meet. There's more. We both hate our new neighborhood; there's too much crime. We've been broken into twice already. Next thing you know our kids will be on drugs. So we're going to move again. And just last week my mother was diagnosed with cancer. She lives 300 miles away. I can't even afford the bus ticket to go visit her. I'm so angry and so depressed. I blame Ted, even though it's not his fault that he lost his job. We fight constantly."

This beleaguered couple, overwhelmed with enormous stress in such a short time, did very well with brief couple's therapy. They had a sound marital infrastructure that had served them well for 15 years. Very soon they each found jobs, their communication got back on track, and so did their sexual relationship.

The Extramarital Affair

An unknown but significant number of marriages go through a crisis because one partner has been unfaithful. These extramarital relationships can be both a cause of and a result of sexual problems in the marriage. Because affairs can be such a complicated issue, this subject will be discussed at length in the next chapter.

FOUR

Extramarital Relationships

Marital covenants carry the expectation of fidelity throughout the life cycle, and most married individuals take their vows very seriously. Therefore, any threat to the sanctity or strength of the marital bond can cause an upset to marital integrity and function.

Before going on, let me make a distinction between the terms *extramarital sex* and *extramarital affair*. Extramarital sex means that the married person has had sex on at least one occasion with someone outside the marriage. Sex may have taken place with little or no feeling for the person at one extreme or with a great deal of feeling and passion at the other. The two individuals may have had sex only once with no expectation or chance of continuity (the "one-night stand"), or they may have had sex several times. What the spouse argues is that it was only sex and not a love relationship, as if that diminishes the sting for his or her partner. Sometimes it does ease the hurt, but the bottom line that must be acknowledged is that this partner has been unfaithful, no matter how it is explained, minimized, or rationalized.

An extramarital affair is a relationship that has developed between a married person and someone outside the marriage. It usually includes sex but not always (even if sex has not occurred, there are usually erotic feelings forming and hopes of consummation at some future point). Affairs usually include loving and affectionate feelings for the other person and a wish to see that individual again and to continue doing so. There is a strong need to be together and an overpowering feeling of being out of control (at least part of the time). There is almost always a fair amount of deception and inner conflict about this, although guilty feelings about the affair vary from one individual to the next.

Voluntary Disclosure

Under what circumstances does a married person tell his or her spouse about being involved with someone else? First, in their marriage they may have agreed to tell each other absolutely everything, no matter how hard or painful it is to do. (Many couples believe they have this kind of openness, but it is usually false—one or both partners often hide an enormous amount from each other.) Second, the one having the affair feels terribly guilty and can't keep it a secret any longer. It now involves a fair amount of lying and fabrication, distortion of events, and omission of fact. In other words, his or her conscience can't bear it and he or she needs the relief that "spitting it out" brings. Third, he or she wants help from the spouse, and by revealing what's going on there is hope of understanding the affair, explaining it, and perhaps ending it. So the person is really turning to his or her spouse for support. Fourth, the person discloses the extramarital relationship because he or she is leaving the marriage to be with the other person. This is usually a mixed blessing for the spouse left behind—it explains why the person wants to separate, but it doesn't accord any opportunity at all to work on the marriage. For those who didn't see the separation coming or even suspect an affair, this can feel like a kick in the stomach.

The above dynamics explain voluntary disclosure and assume a healthy baseline of communication in the marriage. In these circum-stances, it is not unusual for couples who discuss the affair to find that dialogue is helpful. Talking about it may create insight into how the affair began and what to do next—continue the affair or end it.

Discovery

The most common situation is one in which the man's or woman's spouse suspects that there's an affair going on, asks if it's so, is told "No," and within a short period, is told "Yes." Once it's out in the open, they can begin to talk about it and make some decisions about what to do.

Another scenario is one in which people who are having an affair become "careless." They give the impression of setting themselves up to be caught. They might leave credit card receipts around the house, disappear for hours at a time, be absent from work, make mysterious, furtive phone calls, wear clothes with unfamiliar perfume or cologne scents on them, and so forth. These people can't bring themselves to tell the truth about what's really going on and take responsibility for their actions. Individuals who act like this usually have a lifelong pat-tern of behaving passively. They upset those around them with this behavior and with their inaction, as opposed to taking a more ma-ture, responsible, and proactive stance. There is usually other evi-dence of this behavior in the marriage, the workplace, or the family history.

Some individuals don't disclose that they are having an affair and have absolutely no intention, conscious or unconscious, of telling their spouse. They strategically and very carefully plan their outside liaisons, leaving no clues. However, their behavior may seem so inde-pendent or "different" that their spouse becomes suspicious of an affair and begins to plot to catch them. The spouse may even hire a private investigator to check up on his or her partner.

Despite the pain, most people say they would rather be told directly that their husband or wife is having an affair. To have to con-front a deceitful spouse and to have your allegations denied is maddening. To have to become a detective in marriage (or to hire one) is demoralizing. To be told about the affair by "well-meaning" friends is humiliating. To catch your spouse "in the act" creates a wound that never heals.

When the Spouse Doesn't Want to Know

There are some couples in which one of them is having an affair or has had a series of affairs over the years and his or her partner has no knowledge of it. At times friends and acquaintances are aghast at how public the outside relationship may be, and yet the spouse doesn't know or appear to know. One of two possibilities usually explains this. In some marriages, the spouse does know but chooses to live with this fact for a host of reasons: the person married for better and for worse and bears infidelity with courage and dignity; the marriage may function quite well in many other ways and there is a lot of love in many other dimensions of their relationship; there may be a concern about the impact of divorce on their children; there may be a need for financial security; the person may fear being alone; his or her self-esteem may not be very high; or there may be some gratification in being a victim.

The other possibility is denial. In other words, there is a complete inability to see the writing on the wall, that the marriage is in trouble and that there is or could be another person. Denial is a defense mechanism against anxiety and the painful aspects of reality. For some people, facing marital erosion or unhappiness is very frightening or overwhelming—they have to block it out of consciousness even if it is staring them in the face.

What Causes Extramarital Affairs?

I have provided two reasons for the occurrence of extramarital affairs: 1) *individual reasons,* or those that originate within the psyche of the individual (i.e., not caused by an otherwise healthy and functional marriage); and 2) *marital reasons,* or those that stem from within the marriage proper (i.e., problems at home have contributed to the affair). However, these reasons are not necessarily mutually exclusive and in real life will hardly ever be as definite as I've outlined here. There may be a lot of connectedness between individual and marital factors, and they may even be circular; that is, a problem within one person leads to an affair, which then causes a problem in the marriage, which then affects both partners.

Individual Reasons

Immaturity.   In this case, individuals who have affairs haven't yet reached the stage of mature love in their marriages. That is, they are still rather egocentric and self-centered. They may not have very good control over their impulses and can't resist playing out their erotic desires. They are not able to take their marital vows literally.

Inner conflict.   These individuals do not have very high self-esteem and may feel quite insecure about themselves. They may lack sexual confidence and need repeated validation by love, attention, or sex from others.

Alcohol or other drug problems.   In this situation, people lose their normal inhibitions when they are under the influence of alcohol or other drugs. Hence, they may become sexually involved with someone outside the marriage because they are not as careful as they normally would be.

Depression or manic depressive illness (also called bipolar disorder).   When individuals are depressed, they may be more vulnerable to the interest or excitement of someone in their environment who appeals to them. Their mood is so low that it can feel extremely uplifting to be with someone who finds them attractive and intriguing. Because they've been so down at home, their partner may have withdrawn, leaving them feeling abandoned or rejected.

When people are manic (in the manic phase of manic-depressive illness), they feel high, energetic, and sometimes hypersexual. They are prone to extramarital affairs because they are fun and charming and project "sexual energy," and their judgment is skewed; that is, they don't screen people as they normally do and they also "throw caution to the wind." When they are well again, they usually feel ashamed and guilty about their behavior.

Character defect.   In a word, these individuals have long-standing flaws in their personality makeup that may go back to their childhood or adolescence. They are often not honest, and they usually do not have a strong conscience. They are not really capable of a monogamous commitment to one individual and may have a series of "lovers" over the course of their marriage or marriages.

Sexual addiction, compulsive sexuality.   These individuals have a drivenness about them that requires repeated sexual gratification from others, but the relief is not sustained and soon it must be satisfied again with the same partner, or with someone else. Some of these individuals frequently visit prostitutes. In this time of AIDS, they are at high risk for developing HIV disease.

Life-stage factors.   In the chapter "Marriage and the Life Cycle," I give an example of infidelity in the middle years. Midlife is the classic life stage when a man falls in love with someone outside the marriage or has his first affair—the so-called male menopause. However, some individuals may have an affair when they turn 30 or when they turn 40. Whenever it occurs, the individual is usually feeling frustrated or bored with his or her life and is vulnerable to the change and excitement an affair offers.

Job threat or job loss.   Job or career may form a large and important part of one's identity as a human being. "What do you do?" is a common question when strangers meet. If people are laid off or fired, this can be a blow to their self-worth and can render them susceptible to the soothing of someone who really seems to care or understand.

Marital Reasons

The majority of people who find themselves in love with someone other than their spouse are not initially aware of marital difficulty. It is only in the midst of the affair that they begin to think about their marriage in terms of unmet needs or other problems. Some may have been conscious of unhappiness but did not realize how lonely or angry they were in their marriage until they met someone else. A frequent refrain I hear in my office is "I'm not blaming my wife (or my husband) for my affair. I'm just trying to understand how I got involved with someone else."

Of all individuals who do not feel happy in their marriage, some do discuss these feelings with their spouse. If things don't change, with or without professional help, an affair may occur at some time in the future, and it may set a separation process in motion. However, in many marriages, the partners never discuss how unhappy they are—the couple is either blind to the problem or very skilled in hiding unhappiness and seeming fine. These marriages can function quite nicely but emotionally they are fraudulent. If the person begins an affair at some point in the future, the spouse feels shocked and shattered.

Boredom.   Feeling bored in marriage is a common precipitant to starting an affair (because affairs are quite the opposite!). "Is this all there is?" characterizes that state of sameness, predictability, and lack of stimulation that most married people experience at some point in their lives together. If this feeling state corresponds simultaneously with a stage of disillusionment in the marriage, then an affair is possible because the person wonders: "Could I do better with someone else? Do I want to spend the rest of my life with this person?" Boredom, as a dynamic in contributing to an affair, is more common in younger couples than in older. Some couples who have been together a long time say they "can't be bothered having an affair." Or they've seen too many heartaches among family members or friends who have had affairs; or their morality is such that they couldn't; or they have such control over their thoughts, feelings, and impulses that they would never allow themselves to experience exciting feelings for someone else, let alone give in to them.

Loneliness. This is another common emotion in individuals who are having an affair. I think it's as common in men as it is in women, but often men are not as aware as women that they've felt lonely in their marriage. Nor do men talk about feelings of loneliness easily. In my 25 years of listening to couples' problems, I recall very few husbands actually saying "I feel very lonely in my marriage" (as opposed to women, who mention this frequently). However, if I say to a husband who is unhappy and angry, "You seem lonely to me. Are you?" very often he says, "Yes . . . yes, I am."

It is critical to remember the difference between being alone and being lonely. One can be alone and not feel lonely, but one can be not alone and still feel very lonely. This occurs in marriages wherein the two individuals are often together but may not feel connected or supported emotionally. Lonely people are vulnerable to the attention and interests of others. They often don't feel needed, loved, or adored by their spouses. Indeed, they may feel used and taken for granted.

Spouse is "busy." This marital dynamic is often connected with the two previous reasons, in that the person may feel bored or lonely because his or her spouse is so busy with work, the kids, community affairs, and so forth. Many busy people in marriage have no idea how much they are neglecting their partners. They sure find out quickly, however, when they learn of an affair.

Spouse is sick. Married individuals who are ill, especially if they are chronically ill or disabled, are not able to function in a true spousal way. They cannot meet their partners' needs or keep up or do a lot of recreational things. They may not be able to perform usual duties, like hold down a paying job, or help out at home, or even parent. They may not be able to share much of themselves in terms of affection and sex. Their spouses, therefore, feel a responsibility to bear more than their share, which can lead to fatigue or depression and resentment. And if there's no longer much fun in their lives together, an affair may restore this in some ways.

Chronic medical (e.g., brittle diabetes, severe arthritis, ulcerative colitis, multiple sclerosis, severe heart disease, AIDS) and psychiatric (e.g., schizophrenia, refractory depression, severe bipolar illness, drug addiction) disorders that require numerous doctor appointments, hospitalizations, and medications are examples of long-term conditions that can stress a marriage.

Pregnancy or postpartum stage of marriage. Some men begin affairs when their wives are pregnant or in their first postpartum year. These men get involved with someone new because their wives are not able to meet their needs as they once did. Their wives are often preoccupied with being pregnant or are busy with a new and dependent child (and are totally exhausted most of the time). The expectant or new fathers can feel rejected or shoved aside and are vulnerable to the love and attention of others.

Changed sexual relationship in the marriage. For various reasons, couples may find that their sexual relationship has altered, that they do not make love as frequently, that their lovemaking is less satisfying, or that they are really not being honest with

She Says . . .

"My husband never notices when I could use some help around the house. He never takes the initiative; I have to assign him chores."

This woman is upset because she is bearing all, or most, of the responsibility for the maintenance of the home. She may be more than upset (read: angry, resentful, overloaded, bitter); she may also feel sad and frightened. Why? Because in her eyes, her husband doesn't care about her, the marriage, their family.

Perhaps her main concern is that her husband doesn't help with anything that was traditionally defined as "woman's work" (i.e., housework). She has no complaints about the attention he gives to "man's work." We are now talking about a problem of fairness, namely, who does what to get the job done.

But what is central here is that her husband doesn't seem to notice what needs to be done, for example, putting his dishes from an evening snack into the dishwasher or taking out the overflowing garbage. Is she the only one to see what needs to be done? Most of the time, probably yes.

Her husband may be a "work in progress." He is not there yet (he may never be fully there) and is still largely "outer directed." Hence, he doesn't see or hear. In addition, many husbands today have not had these roles modeled for them. They witnessed their fathers doing "more important" work (i.e., paid work outside the home).

Another dimension to this woman's complaint is that she becomes the mother and her husband the child, a transaction that is fraught with all kinds of difficulties. He may indeed hear her, but he is furious and gets back at her by digging in his heels and doing nothing she would like him to do. All of us feel better in our marriages when we relate to our spouses in an adult-to-adult manner.

each other. As one woman said when discussing her marriage: "My husband and I have sex, and I hate it. But my lover and I make love, and I love it." This kind of problem rarely exists in isolation. There are usually other marital dynamics that have contributed to the changed sexual relationship.

Changed intimacy.   This is much more common than a pure change in one's sexual relationship, and it is an especially common complaint of women who start an affair. They complain that their marriage lacks intimacy—warmth, a feeling of closeness, shared purpose, and laughter. Having these needs met by someone other than one's spouse underscores how important they are in marriage. Both women and men need intimacy; however, women are more conscious of "something missing" *before* the affair begins than men.

Other complaints.   Two common examples come to mind. Some individuals start an affair because they say their partner has let him- or herself go. Perhaps they have put on a lot of weight, they pay less attention to their grooming and hygiene, they are not as attractive, or they persist in annoying habits such as smoking. Another example is the situation in which people explain their affair, partly, because their spouse has "gotten old"—they aren't any fun anymore, they have no spontaneity, they are rigid and fixed in their ways, and they are just too conservative. They may simply change or grow apart in their beliefs as the years pass. One of them approaches each life transition with vigor, the other with resignation. A vital connectedness is missing and the gulf between them widens.

The Impact of an Affair

An affair can create a wide range of emotions—from barely a ripple of responsiveness, to catastrophe (including "nervous breakdowns," hospitalization, attempts at suicide, completed suicide, and homicide). There are many factors that determine how people react to the knowledge that their spouse is having an affair.

1. The level of knowledge or suspicion, if any, about the affair. But even if there was some suspicion, the reaction can still be devas-

tating, such as "My worst fear was confirmed when my husband told me that he was in love with his nurse."

2. The amount of denial of possible preexisting marital difficulty. This includes one's ability to examine or reflect on the health or functioning of one's marriage, in other words, one's insight into such an important relationship. Many married people never give their marriage any thought—they just assume it's fine.

3. The degree of trust in one's spouse and whether there was any reason to suspect that he or she could be unfaithful.

4. Whether one was told about the affair directly and openly or whether one discovered it by accident or suspicion.

5. If one was lied to or deceived, especially over time.

6. How much explanation, discussion, and communication occur about the affair once it is out in the open. This can be healing, even if the marriage ends. But if there's no dialogue and the affair is a *fait accompli,* then it's very hard. The spouse just leaves, there is no opportunity to work on the relationship, there is no feedback, and the one left behind is profoundly hurt or profoundly raging.

7. The duration of the affair. This equates with the duration of deception. The longer the deception, which can be years or decades in some marriages, the more the spouse is left wondering, "Was my whole marriage a sham?"

8. The spouse's preexisting health, both physical and mental, can sometimes render the spouse much more wobbly when he or she learns of the affair. Some individuals with a long history of major medical or psychiatric illness cope as well as anyone else under the circumstances. And if their marriage was, in part, aggravating their health, they may actually improve or thrive if their marriage ends in divorce.

The Effect on Marriage
Over the Long Term

Remember—the vast majority of couples beset with an affair do not divorce. There are four major possibilities resultant from extramarital affairs: reconciliation, temporary separation, denial, and separation.

Reconciliation

The couple has a huge marital crisis once the affair is known. They talk and talk and talk; they fight and cry and comfort each other. They make mad passionate love. The outside relationship ends and the marriage is actually strengthened by this crisis. Trust is slowly regained over the next year. The couple may or may not have the assistance of professional help.

Temporary Separation

The couple separates for a few months to a year and then reconciles. The individuals find that the time apart was very fruitful in giving them space—to reflect, to make a decision about the other person, to perhaps receive some individual therapy, to begin to communicate with each other again, to have another courtship with each other before deciding to live together again.

Denial

The couple does not deal at all with the affair—it ends and is not talked about again—nor do the individuals discuss their marriage and any possible problems. In other words, things are swept under the carpet, everyone carries on as if nothing has happened, and the marriage continues. There may be another affair in the future because intrinsic marital problems are never resolved.

Separation

The couple separates and eventually divorces. The outside relationship may or may not continue throughout and after the separation and divorce process. How emotionally devastating this is for the spouse who did not have the affair varies. If the marriage had been in trouble for a long time and both parties were estranged, the affair may simply provide an excuse to separate and divorce. However, if there was little recognition of marital distancing, or if the spouse having the affair is immature, impulsive, or self-centered, then the impact of separation and divorce can be catastrophic. "I had the rug pulled out from under me and I couldn't walk properly for 2 years," one woman said. A man described his experience this way: "What a kick in the gut when my wife left! That was 5 years ago and I'm not over it yet."

Aftermath of an Affair and Reconciliation

The partner who had the affair has to mourn the person with whom he or she fell in love. This may be classic mourning that takes time and is characterized by sadness, longing, pining, crying spells, emptiness, and preoccupation with the person's image. Some partners may be very threatened by the intensity and the duration of this mourning process. They may fear that their spouse will go back on his or her word and leave the marriage after all to be with the other person. Understandably, they want the mourning to be completed as quickly as possible.

When people feel "forced" by their spouse to end the outside relationship to preserve the marriage, they may be bitter and resentful. This is the situation in which the married person had hoped, somewhat irrationally he or she acknowledges, "to have it both ways" or "to have his (or her) cake and eat it too."

Many men who have ended affairs employ the mechanism of compartmentalization to carry on. They forge ahead full throttle as if nothing had happened. They may channel a lot into their work or into sports and they do not want to talk about the affair or be reminded of it. Hence, they react with hostility or dismissiveness when their wives bring up the subject.

The partner who did not have the affair almost always needs to talk about it, to try to understand it, to get centered, to regain a sense of marital security and integrity, to have questions answered, to have doubts assuaged, to make sense of it all, and to understand his or her spouse more deeply, especially his or her conflicts and vulnerabilities. The partner can't trust immediately but needs time, at least a year, especially if there are absences from home and that's how the affair began. The partner worries about it happening again, if not now, much later, in times of stress or adversity. This same spouse needs love, attention, reassurance, and affirmation that his or her partner really wants to remain married. He or she may need to release bottled-up feelings of rage and hurt, and these outbursts may be almost impossible for the spouse to listen to these outbursts and be supportive and reassuring. All in all, it can be a rough road for a while.

Questions

"My wife has just told me that she's having an affair. What should I do?"

REACT! Don't be too understanding! Let yourself experience all of the emotions that are common at a time like this. If you're hurt, say so. If you're sad, cry. If you're furious, get angry. If you're frightened, express your fear. If you blame yourself and feel guilty, say so. And talk and talk and talk until you're exhausted. Try to get some information from your wife. How did this happen? Why? Who is she involved with? Do you know the person? How serious is the relationship?

However, having said this, you must respect your wife's right to withhold certain details that are highly personal, that protect her privacy, and that may hurt you more than you're hurting already. You may need to know details, but you have to weigh whether the information will reassure you or make you feel worse. If you are fortunate, your wife is someone who can appreciate your need to know and will not be withholding for no good reason. There is a case for her disclosing enough detail to explain what is happening and how she is feeling so you can understand.

Even if you are the kind of person who has always believed and stated "If my wife ever cheats on me, she's out the door," don't act impulsively. In fact, don't make any decisions about your marriage until you've had at least a few weeks with this news—to process it, to digest it, to talk about it more with her, to gauge your own reaction, and to monitor hers. Most people are in shock when they first learn that their husband or wife is having an affair. You need time. A lot can happen at this stage, when the affair is out in the open. What seemed like a certainty (and an inevitable separation) may not be so certain the more you talk.

Don't be surprised if talking, fighting, and crying about this leads to a feeling of closeness, returning intimacy, and powerful sex together. It may seem strange to be making love with a woman, your wife, whom you both hate and love simultaneously. However, it is normal to be frightened by this new closeness because you can't gauge its authenticity or continuance. You may feel very vulnerable at the same time, wondering if you're just being used and if your wife doesn't really love you but does love the other man more. So you may long for her and push her away at the same time. And yes, it is normal to worry about AIDS. She has been sexual with someone else, which does introduce another person into your bedroom. Insist on safer sex for 6 months (and HIV-antibody testing) until this is all sorted out, even if your wife thinks you're being "paranoid" and becomes defensive.

Confide in a close and trusted friend or family member who is supportive. You will probably find it essential to tell someone (because you're "bursting" inside) and will feel great relief in getting your thoughts and feelings out. You can "sanitize" what you tell, if it's necessary to protect your wife, yourself, and/or the other person. Make certain whomever you tell will respect your privacy and maintain confidentiality. Don't be surprised if your wife is upset or has mixed feelings that you've confided in someone. She may feel embarrassed and guilty knowing how hard this is for you, and she will worry about being judged. Try to reassure her that you trust the person you've confided in and that he or she is not taking sides.

Pay attention to your general health through this period of uncertainty. You are clearly under extreme stress and may have trouble sleeping, eating, concentrating, remaining in control, not bursting into tears, or not taking your frustrations out on others. If all of this persists, and you are getting run down from not sleeping or eating, see your family physician or internist.

In addition to your feelings (rage, fear, hurt, disbelief, guilt, sorrow), do you also feel a bit sexist about your situation? What I mean is a feeling that men are almost expected to have an affair at some point in their lives whereas women aren't. Do you feel "cuckolded" in a traditional and old-fashioned sense? Do you feel embarrassed that this has happened in your marriage and also feel terribly inhibited about telling anyone, even a close friend or family member whom you really respect and trust? Although the incidence of married men having affairs has always been higher than for married women, this gap is narrowing.

Watch your potential for violence. Even the most mild-mannered of men can become physically aggressive while trying to cope with this type of assault to his marriage, personal security, or masculine self-esteem. Don't bully your wife emotionally or verbally. And if you're not certain, ask your wife if she feels frightened of you, or controlled, or manipulated. On the other hand, you should assert yourself and express what you're feeling, including what you want in terms of your marriage continuing or not. It is essential that you let your wife know exactly what you feel. If you do indeed truly love her (despite how upset you're feeling) and want your marriage to work, say so. She may have had no idea how important she is to you, and this may have played a part in her meeting and falling in love with someone else. Agree to go with her for marital therapy if she is interested and willing. She may not be, arguing that it is too late.

If you and your wife are continuing to be sexually active with each other, pay attention to how you are in bed. More specifically, don't be aggressive, demanding, or punishing in the bedroom. The reason I mention this is because in my practice I have heard many married women who've had an affair complain that their husbands became aggressive in the bedroom. They felt punished in some way. Some have even felt raped by their husbands, although when confronted, their husbands denied these feelings.

Whatever you do, don't go out and have an affair yourself. Any satisfaction you may derive will be short lived, and it won't solve the problem between you and your wife. Likewise, going out and getting drunk may provide some short-term relief, but it isn't really salutary in the long run. You might be prone to violence if you get drunk, and you might end up hurting yourself or someone you don't want to hurt.

To repeat—talk about your feelings, get them out, go to the gym,

open up to a close friend. It helps tremendously to know that someone cares about you while you live through this agonizing time. Pay
attention to your health and see your doctor if you're not coping well.

"I'm not sure if I should trust my husband. Once you've had one
affair, isn't it easier to have another?"

No! Trust your husband—with two provisos. One is that the two of
you have truly talked through the affair and you both understand it,
why and how it happened, that indeed he feels upset about what has
happened and that he understands himself better, and that the two of
you feel much closer as a couple. You should feel confident that you
communicate with each other with more honesty and openness, that
you air grievances, that neither of you shirks from trying to solve problems together. There should be a comfortable sense that your sexual
relationship is back on track or even better than it used to be. You
should have a sense that your marital functioning has been restored.
Trust should be slowly and steadily improving.

Second, make an agreement or contract with each other that if
your husband begins to experience any "warning signals" of an affair
in the future he will tell you about it immediately. This would enable
the two of you to examine what is happening and to discuss what to
do. It might also be a good idea for you to make a similar kind of
promise to him, even if you see yourself as the last person who would
ever have an affair.

"What are the warning signals that I might be heading toward
an affair?"

- Not feeling loved or appreciated at home. There may or may not
  be a change in your sexual relationship.
- Brooding and/or resentment about this.
- Closing off from your spouse and distancing.
- Noticing (more than usual) attractive and interesting individuals
  in your life.
- Beginning to fantasize and/or dream about one or more of these
  people.

- Feeling nervous or excited around these individuals.
- Feeling tempted to act on these thoughts and feelings, or feeling of vulnerable to individuals who seem interested in you.

"I never thought I'd cheat on my wife (or husband). Do you find that hard to believe?"

No, not at all. I hear it almost every day in my work as a psychiatrist and marital therapist. I believe that almost all people take their wedding vows very seriously. Most human beings do not willfully and deliberately set out to cheat on their partner.

Why some people have an affair in response to marital unhappiness or emptiness, as opposed to those individuals who never do, remains a mystery. But I have heard some interesting accounts from my patients and their partners. One man, for example, said to his wife, defensively, after she told him, somewhat self-righteously, that he never had to worry about her having an affair, "No, you just drink!" Other angry outbursts I've heard are "You've just become a couch potato" or "You just overeat" or "All you do is work; work is your mistress." As angry as these responses are, they do get at the heart of the matter. They tap into the underlying marital issues that may have contributed to unhappiness and loneliness, and ultimately to the affair.

Let me reiterate, extramarital affairs are not just about sex. In fact, they may have very little to do with sex. They are about a host of nonsexual needs that aren't being fulfilled in the marriage. And for some couples these are needs that have never been met but were never realized or understood until now.

"I'm worried about my husband. He's 49 years old and having an affair with his secretary. My friends say he's having a midlife crisis. I think it's more serious than that. Could he be depressed?"

Maybe yes—maybe no. Whatever you do, don't ignore what's happening or sweep it under the carpet. Try to talk to him about what's going on in his life and especially his relationship with his secretary. Talk to him as a friend would, if that's possible. It may be possible, despite the hurt you feel about what he's doing or the anger you feel toward him.

Here are some questions you might consider asking yourself in an attempt to understand his actions at the moment. Is he under a lot of pressure at work? Pressure to perform? Is he worried about job security? Is he worried about money and other responsibilities toward the family (despite the fact that he's acting very irresponsibly)?

Is he having trouble with aging? Is he afraid of turning 50?

How has your marriage been the last few months, the last few years? Are the two of you communicating about as well as you normally do? Are you spending much time together as a couple? If so, what's the time like when you're alone as a twosome? How are things in the bedroom?

Is your husband drinking more than usual? How do you feel about this? How's your drinking been lately?

Does your husband seem depressed? Is he irritable, brooding, worried, preoccupied, tense, sad or despondent, sleeping poorly, withdrawn, or tired much of the time? Is he hyper- and overactive, driven, agitated, and unable to sit still? If he is depressed, which came first—the change in his mood or the affair?

How do you feel about all of this? How are you doing? Do you have anyone to talk to for support?

Is your husband confiding in anyone besides you, like a close friend or a member of his family? Encourage him to talk to a professional—his family physician or internist, a psychiatrist or other therapist, or if he's religiously oriented, a member of the clergy.

"My husband (or wife) has been seeing someone else for months now. What should I do?"

You have to think about what you need right now and what you want to see happen. Keep talking with your spouse. Ask yourself how much longer you can live with this situation; consider your personal feelings and circumstances. Matters that can make this difficult are serious financial concerns, young children, a very strong commitment to the notion of family, a strong aversion to separation or divorce, pride, and an image in the community to maintain.

How are things at home overall? Is your marriage not bad except for your partner's affair? How are you coping?

Try to remember that most married people can't live like you are living at the moment. But some can, so you are definitely not alone. You may have to ignore your friends' or family's well-meaning advice to leave. This is your marriage and your decision is ultimately your own. And it is a decision of the heart (what *feels* right for you) and not a decision of the brain (what you *think* you should do).

If you've come to the conclusion that you can't stand it any longer, here are some options:

1. Give your spouse a deadline of, say, 6 weeks to 3 months to end the outside relationship, after which you'll have to have a separation if the affair has not ended. You must be prepared to stick by your guns if he or she doesn't end the affair.
2. Announce right now that you want to separate, and launch into negotiations—who will move out and when, how and when to tell the children, interim financial arrangements, and so forth.
3. Insist on marital therapy together.
4. Get some individual psychotherapy for yourself to help you through this ordeal. The support of someone outside your network of friends or family can be invaluable, especially when you are not able to see how far you've come in terms of your improved self-esteem, emerging independence, strength, and assertiveness.

FIVE

Excessive Drinking in Marriage

Problem drinking is one of the most common complaints in marriage. It is estimated that there are 10 million adult alcoholics in the United States, and a large number of those individuals are or have been married. It is a problem for both genders but much more common in men than in women.

When couples come for marital therapy with alcohol as a concern, there are one of two patterns—the excessive drinking stands alone as the issue or drinking is merely one of several marital complaints. In the former, one partner is blamed by his or her spouse for the marriage faltering. "If my husband would only stop drinking, things would be fine. He's quit before, for 2 years, and we were happy. Since he returned to the bottle, we've all been miserable." This may not be the whole story, but it is perceived or conceptualized this way by the nondrinking spouse and other family members.

In the second pattern, drinking is one of several concerns, as in the following statement:

> Oh, we've got a lot of problems—we've never communicated very well, so we fight a lot, usually over silly stuff. My mother's been really sick the past 4 years and living with us; that's a lot of extra work for my

wife, which she resents. Our son got arrested for drug trafficking and he may be going to jail. Our 14-year-old daughter is pregnant—she dropped out of school. I was laid off last year—I couldn't find work for 9 months. We had to move into a rented home in a neighborhood that we hate. My wife was in an accident last year and her back is all messed up so she can't go back to work—she's a practical nurse—and to make matters worse, she's been hitting the bottle pretty heavy. We fight a lot about that. I think she's on her way to becoming an alcoholic—everyone else in her family is—but she thinks I'm blowing it way out of proportion.

The Effect of Alcohol on Marriage

Alcohol has an extremely negative effect on marriage and the family. It is actually a family disease in that drinking in one person affects everyone and they, in turn, affect the drinking pattern. Alcoholism in families renders them dysfunctional in many respects:

- Family members don't communicate with each other
- They don't respect or support each other
- There is mistrust among family members
- Responsibility for chores and tasks in the home is not shared easily or comfortably
- Family members don't laugh and enjoy each other very much
- They don't share meals, conversation, and leisure
- There are not very many family traditions, rules, rituals, or honoring of each other
- There are many family secrets and people can become quite isolated, not only from each other but from others outside the family
- There is tremendous shame

In many alcoholic families there are rules that are never openly stated but that exist nonetheless. The most dysfunctional person, the alcoholic, makes the rules, which are the following:

1. The use of alcohol is the most important thing in the family's life. It doesn't have to be stated, it just is.

2. Someone or something else caused the alcohol dependency; the alcoholic is not to blame. It's stress. It's unemployment. It's in the family.

3. The status quo must be maintained at all costs. The family will continue on as it always has.

4. Everyone in the family must be an enabler. All family members contribute in some way to the continuation of the drinking pattern in the alcoholic by defending him or her, making excuses, covering up, or actually buying the alcohol.

5. No one may discuss what is really going on in the family, either with one another or especially with outsiders.

6. No one may say what he or she is really thinking or feeling. "Let's pretend that everything is fine."

In some alcoholic families, certain roles are assigned or assumed by family members: the spouse becomes the Chief Enabler and the children become the Hero, the Scapegoat, the Lost Child, or the Mascot. The labels speak for themselves and serve to highlight how each of these roles has its own pain, function, and payoffs in a family disease process such as alcoholism.

Various Drinking Patterns

There are definite drinking patterns that defy society's stereotype of the alcoholic. This is partially the reason that some alcoholic individuals and their family members so defensively deny that a problem exists. There is a belief that unless the person who drinks is falling-down drunk every day and can't hold down a job because of drunkenness, that person is not an alcoholic. Well, that picture shows only one type of alcohol problem, albeit the most visible and obvious kind. There are many others: people who drink daily but only after work and who have "never missed a day's work" or "who never drink before work" or "on the job." Some individuals only drink on the weekends—but are literally under the influence of alcohol from Friday night at 5 P.M. until they go to bed Sunday night. Their behavior shows it because they are not very functional in terms of getting anything done or interacting in any meaningful way with their families or friends on weekends, which are often set aside for family and social activities. These people will also use holidays as a reason to drink. Some are binge drinkers; that is, they go for days or weeks literally drinking nonstop, except when they're passed out, and they tend to drink until they become medically or psychiatrically ill and/or their money runs out. But between alcoholic binges, they either don't drink a drop or drink only socially.

What is most important from the perspective of the family is not so much the pattern of use but how alcohol affects the feelings of family members. And this is where behavior is significant, because alcohol changes one's behavior, even though people who drink tend to minimize or deny this. How can the chorus of millions of spouses and kids of alcoholic parents throughout the world be wrong? They all say the same thing, that their spouse or their mom or dad changes with alcohol and becomes withdrawn, sleepy, touchy, sarcastic, provocative, abusive, violent, unpredictable, maudlin, despairing, pathetic, silly, inappropriate, disinhibited, embarrassing, garrulous, or forgetful. Need I say more?

The attitude toward drinking is a big factor in determining whether someone thinks there's a problem. Our attitudes about drinking are affected by our culture, ethnic heritage, religious beliefs or lack thereof, and family values. There is a continuum from very

---

He Says . . .

"My wife is a wonderful woman. I just wish she wouldn't nag me so much."

We reveal a lot about ourselves when we complain about our spouses and in how we word our complaints. This man should ask, "What does my complaint about my spouse tell me about myself?"

What does he mean by "nagging"? When asked to elaborate, he may say, "She is always on my case—she never lets up—I don't get a moment to relax." When asked how he feels about this, he might say, "Feel? Well, I don't like it. She makes me angry and then I resent her. She treats me like one of our children. It's demeaning."

I could say to him, "Do you think that maybe you do behave like a child sometimes?" Or I might ask, "Is there anything that you do or don't do that brings out so-called nagging in your wife?" Both questions are provocative and intended to make him think about the parent-child transactional nature of "nagging."

conservative and negative attitudes toward alcohol in any form at one extreme to very liberal and accepting attitudes at the other. Within marriage it's not unusual for the drinking person to defend and rationalize his or her drinking because of the spouse's judgment and intolerance.

Finally, it is not actually the specific amount of alcohol the person drinks that is so upsetting to the spouse but what alcohol does to the relationship. As a marital therapist I find I can be much more helpful to the couple who has come to see me if I don't get embroiled in determining whether the amount of alcohol consumed warrants a diagnosis of alcoholism. My job is to point out what the use of alcohol *seems* to be doing to marital harmony and solidarity.

How Does Alcohol Affect Marriage?

Let me start with some positives, because there are some, for those people who do drink and who enjoy it in a healthy way. First, there is the relaxation effect of alcohol that seems especially welcome after a long or busy day. It's implicit in the statements "Come in and sit down and we'll have a drink together" or "Let's split a bottle of wine with dinner." Second, there is the celebratory effect, part of toasting with a flute of champagne: "Happy anniversary, dear." Third is the euphoriant properties of alcohol: "I feel good, I feel happy, I feel wonderful being married to you." Fourth, alcohol in small amounts promotes conversation: "You're a lot more talkative since having that scotch before dinner . . . I like that." Fifth, alcohol is disinhibiting: "I have to admit that I do feel a lot more affectionate and interested in sex when I've had a small glass of wine."

Now for the negatives. Unfortunately, there are a lot of these.

1. Alcohol depresses the central nervous system; that is, it makes us sleepy, listless, or despondent. It's hard to communicate with your spouse or other members of your family if you feel any of the above.
2. Most spouses are turned off by alcohol on the breath of someone they're in a relationship with. This is a negative consequence

that causes one's partner or spouse to pull away or get depressed or angry. Again, this affects good feeling and harmony and may ruin any possibility of close affection, including making love.

3. Alcohol is also a disinhibiting chemical—it loosens or removes our usual inhibitions. Hence, some people become sarcastic, mean, irritable, argumentative, overtalkative, or violent. Some of the worst fights and arguments I hear about from the couples who come to see me are related to one or both of them drinking too much. They are at risk for physical assaultiveness toward each other and their children. It is also known that at least some instances of sexual abuse of children occur under the influence of alcohol.

4. Alcohol affects us sexually. Some men cannot get erections or ejaculate as usual. Some women lose interest in sex or can't have orgasms. Some people become quite seductive or sexually aggressive when they've had a lot to drink. Some people get sexually demanding or rough in bed with too much alcohol.

5. Alcohol can affect a person's social behavior. He or she may flirt with other individuals at parties or become sexually inappropriate. Behavior may become controlling. Jokes that are told are not appropriate or are off-color. Someone who is the so-called life of the party may actually have an edge to his or her behavior; not all participants find the person charming or entertaining. Alcohol can also cause people to withdraw at parties or pass out or vomit. Again, none of these behaviors are particularly endearing to a spouse or partner.

6. There are many changes in the way people communicate under the influence of alcohol. People don't communicate clearly in a progressive and mutually engaging dialogue when they are drunk. They may be touchy, and certain areas of sensitivity must be avoided at all costs. The person usually can't concentrate very well, so things have to be repeated, to the annoyance of spouses, partners, and other family members. Alcohol also affects memory, so many things that were discussed are not remembered the next day. Some people cannot solve problems with their spouses if alcohol is involved, whereas others don't even try because they have no will to discuss anything other

than the most mundane or superficial topics.

7. Nondrinking partners in marriage usually begin to feel left out, abandoned, and resentful of the bottle. They begin to feel, usually quite accurately, that they are secondary. When an alcohol problem is entrenched and serious, alcohol is foremost in the drinker's mind. The spouse becomes incidental or taken for granted.

8. Alcohol affects our bodies and often the physical changes are not pretty. Alcoholics often look older than their age, like they've "been around" and life has not treated them kindly. They are less attractive and physically appealing than they used to be. Men may develop a "beer belly," whereas women may also put on weight around their waist. Both sexes can appear bloated and can develop a ruddy complexion.

9. Damage to one's health also affects marriage. People who are dependent on alcohol may develop ulcers, pancreatitis, and liver disease. From a mental health perspective, they may develop paranoia and begin to think they are being threatened or harmed by a range of known or unknown enemies. They may experience DTs (delirium tremens), alcoholic hallucinosis (hearing very frightening and threatening voices), or alcoholic dementia (similar to Alzheimer's disease).

10. With this kind of damage to physical and mental health, many alcohol-dependent people can't work, or they may be fired because of absenteeism or risks to safety (e.g., airline pilots, train operators, physicians, nurses). In certain cases the person may be sued because of a mishap at work, exacerbating the downward spiral of financial security. The healthy partner in the marriage becomes the primary or sole wage earner or the caretaker of the ill spouse at home. There may be much sorrow and resentment about what has happened to a marriage that was once happy and healthy. There is a strong possibility of separation and divorce anywhere along this chain of events.

11. Alcoholic drinking becomes learned behavior for the children, who are already at risk for alcoholism because of genetic transmission. This is particularly serious because of the cycle of pathological drinking passing from one generation to the next.

When Drinking Becomes a Problem

If you're wondering if you drink too much, then you probably do! Perhaps that's not fair, but what I mean is, it's good that you're asking the question. If you're questioning yourself or your spouse early enough, you can monitor your drinking and cut back on your consumption of alcohol, drastically if necessary.

How much people drink is so subjective and so influenced by cultural and familial factors that what is normal social drinking for Fred may be pathological drinking for Tom. I encourage people who wonder if they're drinking excessively to try cutting down, if they haven't already. As one man recently said to me, "I decided I was drinking too much. I was having one or two drinks every night of the week. So I stopped drinking during the week, unless I'm out at a social function, and even then I may just have mineral water. I only really drink now on weekends and I'm really watching that too. I feel a lot better for it. And I'm relieved that I can control it because I really love a drink. I would hate to have to give it up completely because I'm an alcoholic."

I suggest to people of all ages that they try to cultivate a personal attitude of health-promoting vigilance, that they watch their alcohol use the same way that they watch their diet, their exercise, and their leisure time. By doing this they are really and truly treating alcohol as a drug that must be treated with respect. With this kind of mind-set, they can then gauge if they are drinking too much, just as they can tell if they are not watching their diet properly and gaining too much weight.

Another response to the question of whether you're drinking too much is "If someone who cares about you is more worried about your drinking than you are, they are probably right. You have something to be worried about." When people have alcoholism, their ability to deny the reality of their addiction or to rationalize their drinking is absolutely profound. It has nothing to do with intelligence, education, or knowledge about alcoholism. It is part of the disease itself.

There are lists of classic symptoms of alcoholism (e.g., craving, increasing tolerance, hangovers, morning shakes, memory lapses, blackouts), available in many different publications for the public.

But I always advise people who are worried about their drinking, or someone else's, not to get too focused on whether they have "enough" of the classic symptoms. Go by your gut feeling. And if you don't know for sure, just stop drinking for 1 to 3 months and see if you feel better and if your relationship or marriage has improved (or at least feels more interesting and stimulating).

What Causes Alcoholism?

In addition to what I've touched on above, alcoholism has been called the most "untreated treatable disease" in America today. There is no single cause. But it *is* a disease—one that is both biogenetic (it has physical features and is inherited from one generation to the next) and psychosocial (it has psychological and social causes and effects). It is a disease that has a known cause (too much ethyl alcohol), attacks most organs of the body, changes one's body chemistry, has a predictable and progressive course, and, without intervention, is often fatal.

There is a set of recognizable signs and symptoms characteristic of alcoholism: the person keeps drinking despite adverse and sometimes lethal consequences; there is destruction of one's physical health; there is destruction of one's mental health; there is destruction of one's social, spiritual, and cultural life; the person's tolerance of alcohol changes so that small quantities really affect the person, or the other way around—the person has to drink larger quantities of alcohol to feel its effects; if the person stops drinking, there is a characteristic withdrawal reaction that is very unpleasant and frightening; and the person experiences blackouts or amnesia (there is no memory for recent events).

What to Expect From Your Doctor

Physicians encounter patients every day who suffer, either directly or indirectly, from substance use disorders, including alcoholism. In addition, increasing numbers of family physicians and internists follow the guidelines of (or are certified by) the American Society of Addiction Medicine, the members of which have developed a rigorously tested body of scientific and clinical knowledge about chemical dependency. Therefore, you can expect most or all of the following from your doctor.

Your physician will conduct a thorough medical history and physical examination. This will include many questions about your use of alcohol and any other drugs (including over-the-counter drugs, caffeine, tobacco, street drugs, and prescription drugs). Some of the questions will be about how alcohol affects you and if it changes your behavior or causes a loss of control. Your doctor may also ask about any other compulsive behaviors like excessive exercising, overeating, dieting, sexual obsessiveness, gambling, excessive shopping, shoplifting, and so forth. You will be asked about your family, both current and past, and specifically about its use of alcohol and other drugs. Your doctor will also ask about your mental functioning and he or she may test your mood, your thinking processes, memory, judgment, and problem-solving ability. It is important to see if you have symptoms of a psychiatric disorder (or a history of mental illness in you or your family) because sometimes people with a drinking problem are not aware of this. Your family doctor may wish to talk to your partner or spouse to gain any additional information about your drinking and its effects on others.

You will have laboratory investigations to screen for any damage to your body or changes in your blood or body chemistry. You may have blood or urine tests for alcohol and other drugs.

Your physician should be able to make a tentative diagnosis and will explain his or her findings and impressions to you and perhaps your partner or spouse.

The treatment recommendations made to you may involve a number of health professionals and different types of treatment. Much will depend on your doctor's experience with chemical dependency and the specifics of your situation. Examples include detoxification and residential treatment in a specific setting established for the treatment of alcohol and drug illness; Alcoholics Anonymous (AA); Alanon for your partner or spouse; Alateen for your children; regular counseling by a specialist in alcohol and drugs; group therapy; couples therapy; individual treatment by a psychiatrist, especially if you have an associated psychiatric illness such as depression, obsessive-compulsive disorder, or posttraumatic stress disorder.

Your doctor will not want you to take or be prescribed any medications that are habit forming or addictive. Examples include most tranquilizers, most sleeping pills, and painkillers that include narcotics such as codeine, meperidine (Demerol), and morphine. Excepted drugs are antidepressants, aspirin, and acetaminophen (Tylenol).

Your physician will be interested in how you are doing and will make an effort to coordinate the various kinds of programs that you may be attending. His or her approach to you should be compassionate and kind but also firm and confrontational if you are not able to see or accept the obvious impact of your illness on you or your loved ones.

Dual Diagnosis

If your doctor says you have a "dual diagnosis," you have a drinking problem *plus* an associated or underlying psychiatric illness. Some examples are anxiety disorder, panic disorder, obsessive-compulsive disorder, posttraumatic stress disorder, anorexia nervosa, bulimia, clinical depression ("chemical depression"), and bipolar disorder (used to be called manic-depressive illness). It's very possible that you have camouflaged the psychiatric illness with alcohol so that it's masked or changed in some way. It's also possible that the symptoms and emotional pain of mental illness have caused you to drink or at least have contributed to your drinking so much. In other words, you have been using alcohol to try to calm your nerves or to pick you up if you've been feeling down. Because alcohol is a depressant, you've inadvertently made yourself feel worse.

Your doctor probably also asked you about your family background. This is because alcoholism and many psychiatric disorders run in families. You may have a number of relatives whom you would call alcoholic, but it is possible that some of them might have had a psychiatric problem that was never diagnosed and properly treated. So they treated themselves, so to speak, with alcohol. We know a lot more about mental illness today than we knew a generation ago.

When individuals have a dual diagnosis it means that simply stopping drinking alcohol and receiving drug-free treatment may not be enough to get feeling better again. In fact, there is a risk of slipping back into drinking if the psychiatric illness is not treated. This is because the severe anxiety symptoms, panic, compulsive rituals, bingeing and starving, or feelings of despair are so overwhelming they are impossible to live with.

Your doctor then may suggest a range of treatments, in addition to treatment for your alcoholism, for the symptoms of the other illness. These may be an antidepressant drug, an antiobsessional drug, a sedative for your anxiety—but only drugs that are not habit forming or addictive. Other treatments for symptoms are cognitive therapy, behavior therapy, supportive psychotherapy, group therapy, and marital or family therapy, depending on the specifics of your situation.

Which Comes First?

Does alcohol cause marital discord or do marital problems cause problem drinking? Both are true, but the former is much more common than the latter. A large number of marriages are destroyed each year because of excessive drinking by one or both parties. Many, if not most, of these marriages end in separation and divorce. And unfortunately, it is only at this point, for some alcoholics, that they are able to see how ravaging and damaging their illness really is. If the person accepts treatment at the point of separation, his or her sobriety may become a bargaining chip in whether the parties reconcile. For some spouses, however, even though their husband or wife receives and embraces treatment for alcoholism, it is too late. There is irreparable damage to the couple's love, mutual respect, trust, affection, and solidarity. Permanent separation or divorce is the only option.

Two Examples of Drinking in Marriage

Bill and Gloria

Bill began drinking fairly heavily when he was an undergraduate at college. In fact, it wasn't unusual for Bill to get drunk when he and

Gloria were just dating. They were popular and outgoing. Most of Bill's drinking was "party" drinking, and he had fairly good control over it. He would stop drinking if Gloria thought he had had enough.

Bill and Gloria got married after a courtship of 3 years, when Bill was a second-year dental student and Gloria had graduated and was working at the university as an administrative assistant to a faculty member. During her first pregnancy, which began in Bill's final year of dental school, he began to drink quite a lot, but he cut back a bit after the baby was born. After their second child was born 3 years later, Bill began to have a few beers every day after work, before and during dinner. His weekend drinking also increased in amount and intensity. He would have memory lapses, and Gloria invariably drove home from any parties they attended together.

On Bill's 33rd birthday he was charged with impaired driving, after a late poker game and some very heavy drinking with friends. Over the next several months he and Gloria began to fight more often. She locked him out one night and told him not to return unless he stopped drinking. He did and Gloria took him back a week later. Things were fine for about a month. But when his drinking returned, as regular as ever, Gloria insisted on marriage counseling. Bill agreed. He came to the first visit after a few beers. Gloria was furious. He refused to return to the counselor. One month later Bill moved back home to live with his parents, both of whom were heavy drinkers. However, Bill began attending AA and a support group for dentists with drug and alcohol problems. He stopped drinking for 3 months. He and Gloria reconciled again. He kept attending AA, and Gloria went to Alanon. However, after a year, both admitted that they were only staying together for the children. When Bill met someone in his AA group, he and Gloria separated again. They divorced 3 years later.

Allen and Mary

Allen and Mary were both 40 years old and lived a comfortable, albeit busy, two-professional marriage. Allen was the CEO of a major mining company, Mary the principal of a private girls school. They had three children and were assisted by a full-time nanny.

As Allen became busier at work (more and more responsibility at the office, longer working days, early morning meetings, weekend retreats, and overseas travel), Mary became increasingly lonely and unhappy with her life. She began having a glass of wine before dinner while waiting for Allen to come home. Soon she was having two glasses. Within a year she found herself drinking "a bit" of cognac at bedtime. As Allen's work took him away from home more and more often, Mary met a man through a board on which she served. He loved martinis. Their 3-month affair centered around conversation, drinks, and sex. After a while, Allen confronted her about her unexplained absences and she told him about the man she was seeing.

It was at this point that they came for marital therapy. Mary ended her affair, and with my encouragement she went to AA. Allen agreed to major reshuffling of his work responsibilities so that he could be home more. Within months their relationship was flourishing.

Some Final Questions

"**I** left my husband last week and told him that our marriage is over unless he stops drinking. I still really love him. Do you think I made a mistake?"

No! Obviously you have reached a point where you can't take it anymore. My hunch is that you have been concerned about his drinking for some time, but he hasn't heard you when you've tried to discuss it. This is the massive denial associated with alcoholism. Some alcoholics do not "see the light" until their spouse has left. By your leaving, you have given your husband a very clear message: "You have a serious illness that is ruining our marriage and pulling me down. I now need to take care of myself. Get treatment. Then we will see what's left of our relationship." So hold your ground. Wait and see if you can trust his motivation to make important changes in his life.

Here are some other suggestions:

1. Go to Alanon if you are not attending already.
2. Don't have any contact with your husband if he is still drinking, except for emergencies. If you have children, and you worry about their safety under his care, do not allow visitation. This may require a court order, but you must be at peace with yourself.

3. If your husband does seek help—sees his doctor, goes to detox, attends AA, accepts alcohol and drug counseling—encourage him from a distance.
4. Insist on absolute sobriety for at least 3 months, unless a health professional who is a specialist in alcoholism deems him a controlled drinker, that is, capable of returning to and respecting the social use of alcohol.
5. At that point, if you are both interested and willing, you should consider a gradual and carefully paced courtship.
6. Do not impulsively reconcile, irrespective of how lonely each of you or one of you feels or how determined you are to reunite the family for the sake of your children. They will be better in the long run to grow up with parents who live apart than with parents who are miserable together.
7. Be patient—with him and yourself.

"**M**y wife is drinking more and more. When I come home from work, there's no dinner and she's passed out. She won't admit that she has a problem and she won't go to our doctor or to a counselor. What can I do?"

Start by analyzing your own feelings about her drinking. Make certain that you are not inadvertently reinforcing your wife's illness by bringing alcohol into the home or drinking with her. Many husbands do this because of their naiveté about addiction ("I can control my drinking, why can't you?"), their codependency, and their complete inability to communicate how deeply upset they are about the drinking. From what you're saying, you sound quite concerned—and powerless. I suggest that you give up drinking yourself. Try to discuss the problem with a family member or a close friend. Whatever you do, don't ignore the problem. It won't go away on its own. Be supportive of your wife, but firm. Be aware that she will deny or minimize her drinking (it's part of the illness), but don't you get drawn in by her excuses.

I also suggest that you begin attending Alanon meetings in your community. You'll meet others whose spouses have a problem with drinking. Don't be deterred that there will be very few husbands or partners of women with alcoholism at Alanon. Because alcoholism is more common in men than women, quite naturally there will be more women in Alanon than men. In addition to that, many husbands of alcoholic women, despite their worry and concern, do not reach out for help (like men in general). They try to go it alone. You will benefit from the supportive and caring atmosphere in addition to the program itself. Let your wife know where you are going.

What about going to see an alcohol and drug counselor yourself? He or she will assess your own drinking pattern and how you respond to the problem in your wife. This person will also ask you about your wife's illness and should be able to give you a rough idea of how serious the problem is and some options. There may be a number of possibilities that you haven't considered. One of these might be an intervention wherein you and other family members and one or more professionals confront your wife in your home about the problem. At that time, she may be escorted to an alcohol detoxification center that includes residential treatment for at least a month after detox. This will be the beginning of a comprehensive assessment and treatment plan conducted by a range of health professionals.

At some point in her rehabilitation, when she has been abstinent and in recovery for a while, it might be wise for the two of you to have some marital therapy. The goal would be to assist with a redefinition of your marriage. The drinking has caused both of you to be in certain unhealthy roles with each other for so long that it will be necessary to relate to each other in healthier and more mature ways. You may also need to rediscover each other, regain trust, and work on intimacy, both emotionally and sexually. A marital therapist can assist with this.

References

Griner ME, Griner PF: Alcoholism and the family, in Alcoholism: A Guide for the Primary Care Physician. Edited by Barnes HN, Aronson MD, Delbanco TL. New York, Springer-Verlag, 1987, pp 159–166

Milhorn HT Jr: Chemical Dependence: Diagnosis, Treatment, and Prevention. New York, Springer-Verlag, 1990, pp 79–95

Talbott GD: Alcoholism and other addictions: a primary disease entity. Journal of the Medical Association of Georgia 75:490–494, 1986

Wegscheider-Cruse S: The family disease, in Another Chance: Hope and Health for the Alcoholic Family. Edited by Wegscheider S. Palo Alto, CA, Science and Behavior Books, 1981, pp 76–103

SIX

Psychiatric Illness and Marriage

We've come to one of the most important chapters in this book. Why? I say this because there is an intricate relationship between personal mental health and marital health.

First, here are a few facts and general comments. Psychiatric illnesses are common in our society, despite the fact that they tend to get split off from general medical disorders by the lay public and the insurance industry as less worthy of attention and reimbursement. Misconceptions abound—psychiatric disorders are self-induced, self-indulgent, and untreatable; they are a sign of weakness, incompetence, or moral failing; and we should be suspect of anyone who has been treated for psychiatric illness, especially if he or she is in a position of some importance and responsibility. No wonder, then, that fighting against the stigma associated with psychiatric illness plays such an important role in the professional calling of psychiatrists.

When a married person suffers from a psychiatric illness, he or she is more prone to marital distress, conflict, and marital breakdown than someone who doesn't have this type of illness. Please consider that statement for a moment. Place it in the context of knowing that *most* couples suffer from marital conflict at times and that separation and divorce are very common in North America. Roughly 40% to 50% of people marrying today will divorce. I want you to get a sense of how at risk a married person can feel when he or she has a psychiatric illness.

We also know that in a certain percentage of couples *both* partners have psychiatric disorders. So this makes their lives together feel even more precarious. It's hard to be a "good" husband or wife when you don't feel well, when you're depressed, when you're intoxicated from alcohol, when you're agoraphobic, when you have obsessive-compulsive disorder and have to wash your hands 100 times a day. When both marriage partners are afflicted with psychiatric illness, they are rarely ill at the same time. One of them will be stable and doing well during the period that the other is unwell, so sometimes he or she can provide support and take over responsibilities at home and in the workplace. Because I am both a psychiatrist and a marital therapist, it is not unusual for me to have one or both of the marriage partners on medication and to do marital therapy as well.

Marital unhappiness and conflict can affect your mental health. That is, marital strain can make you sick. Most of the time this is very obvious. For example, you know that you feel depressed because you're so unhappy in your marriage, that you can't sleep because you're worried about your marriage, that you're having panic attacks because your wife is out with her boyfriend, that you've lost 20 pounds since you found out your husband is bisexual, that you're drinking much more since your husband raped and beat you.

But sometimes marital dysfunction is more subtle and only a friend, a family member, or a professional can see that you're feeling the way you are because of a problem at home. If you've been told over and over that you're "frigid," you believe it if you have no other experience to the contrary. You will need to be told that perhaps you are sexually unresponsive because you don't feel loved, or you don't trust your husband, or that your husband is rough with you and not a gentle, sensitive lover.

If you were criticized and put down a lot while you were growing up, you may see this treatment as normal. Consequently, you may not notice how much you are being taken for granted by your husband or wife, how often you are scolded, how much your opinions don't matter, and how much your self-esteem has been eroded through the course of your years together. You internalize all of this and don't speak up in an assertive way or defend yourself. You may prefer to "keep the peace," or you may fear your spouse's wrath if you do challenge or pose a counterargument. This process can make you prone to depression or various physical illnesses that can be stress related, such as asthma, arthritis, low back pain, and headaches.

Communication in some marriages is so dishonest that a person may feel that he or she is going crazy. This is a terrifying experience. The following is an example from my practice.

Frank and Linda

For months, while he was undergoing chemotherapy for cancer, Frank suspected that his wife Linda was having an affair with a co-worker. He brought up the subject often; Linda would reassure him that she was working late on various documents with David but that their relationship was "strictly business." Frank would be fine for a few weeks but then something would occur that made him feel insecure again and would rekindle his suspicions: a couple of phone calls where the caller hung up when he answered; a credit card receipt for a dinner in a restaurant that he and Linda had never been to together; a certain distance and defensiveness in Linda that he had never experienced in his 10 years of marriage to her. Whenever he discussed all of these things with her, she denied anything untoward and showered him with attention (and sex) so he'd feel better again—for a while.

Frank began to feel that he was "going loony." He couldn't sleep, he lost weight, he was obsessed with his marriage, and he became more despondent. He wondered if it was the chemotherapy that was making him mistrustful and panicky. Even worse, he wondered if the cancer might have spread to his brain. He asked his oncologist about this, without mentioning specifics, and he was told that he was doing very well from a medical standpoint and not to worry. When more and more "mysterious" things happened, Frank decided to talk to a long-standing friend about going to see a psychiatrist. His friend listened carefully and compassionately. He said, "You don't need a shrink. You need a detective!" And this is what Frank did. He hired a detective, his suspicions were confirmed, he confronted Linda, she confessed, they each hired divorce attorneys, and they separated.

Not all individuals with moderate or severe marital discord develop psychiatric symptoms. In fact, many develop a range of physical symptoms that cause them to see their physicians. The doctors look for and weigh the various factors that might be causing the illness biologically (e.g., genetic, molecular, bacterial, viral, biochemical, immunological factors), psychologically (e.g., unhappy early home life, strained marriage, poor self-esteem, limited coping resources, depression), and socially (e.g., isolation, economic deprivation, racial/ethnic discrimination, unemployment, recent immigration). Even if the person has very clear and significant high blood pressure, it is not enough merely to treat this with medication. One has to evaluate his or her diet, personal habits like smoking and drinking, the amount of stress in his or her daily life, and how much the person expresses psychological distress through his or her body. Some individuals of certain ethnocultural groups would not necessarily feel depressed when their spouse begins drinking again after 2 years of sobriety. But their colitis sure acts up . . . or their gout . . . or their prostatitis.

Whatever the connection between psychiatric illness and marital discord, whether people get ill because of their marriages or their illness strains their marriage, it's a very hard road. Although we have come a long way toward acceptance of life stressors over the past several decades, there is still a certain amount of stigma associated with seeing a psychiatrist, seeing a marriage therapist, or getting a divorce. Individuals struggle with feelings of failure and seem ashamed in the eyes of their friends and families. No wonder many people remain in loveless or dysfunctional marriages, sometimes forever. This is exemplified in one woman's statement to me: "No, I'm not going to leave this empty marriage. Why broadcast my failure? Dealing with my own conscience is all I can handle, thank you. Let me live the facade."

Another general comment concerns communication. Communication in marriage is central and is the hallmark of marital integrity and function. Communication problems are probably the most common complaint of troubled couples—certainly, marriage therapists hear this day in and day out. Communication facility also is the bedrock or substrate in most marriages. Indeed, many individuals believe that good communication is the great equalizer and the key to sorting out all kinds of marital struggles. Many people actually say this in so many words: "We've always prided ourselves on our ability to communicate; this is why we're so desperate for help right now; we can't talk about the weather without screaming at each other." Or, "Now that we're able to communicate with each other, to talk things through, to really get below the surface, we don't need to come for marital therapy anymore. We can work through this great list of problems on our own over time." Or, "Sure, I'm devastated that we're both HIV positive, but now that we can talk about this awful mess with each other and not blitz out on drugs all the time, I think we'll be OK."

It's very hard to communicate effectively when you're not feeling well, when you're

She Says, He Says . . .

She says: "I love him but he drives me nuts. He's obsessed with sex."

He says: "I wish she'd get horny once in a while. I'm always the one to bring up sex, and most of the time she's just not interested."

Rarely is this the whole story or even an accurate representation of what the woman's husband feels. Very few men are "obsessed with sex," but a lot of men aren't happy with the frequency of sexual activity. What appears to be a preoccupation is actually verbal or behavioral attempts to make physical contact. Unfortunately, many of these efforts are feeble, overstated, oblique, repeated ad nauseam, and off the mark.

Sometimes men are playing a societal role (aren't all men, from adolescence to old age, supposed to have sex on their minds?). A seeming obsession with sex can also be indicative of a fear that their sexuality is waning, that time is flying by and they're not getting any younger. Or it is a sense of entitlement. They got married with the expectation that sex would be on a regular basis and it would be mutual.

Most women experience sexual desire on a regular basis, but it is usually more subtle and highly associated with feelings of love, security, trust, and relaxation. This is not to say that women don't have purely lusty sexual urges—of course they do—but few express these desires in the ways that men think they should.

It is too bad that so often couples get stuck at the physical level and become polarized: he comes to see her as sexually flawed and, consequently, she feels criticized and put down as sexually inadequate; she begins to see her husband as obsessed with sex and, consequently, he feels diminished and further rejected.

exhausted, depressed, manic, inebriated, overwhelmed with anxiety or panic, or bulimic and bingeing and purging. It's also hard when you're from a background with poor communication patterns, when nonverbal communication overshadows verbal, when violence rules, or when you're affected with dementia and your ability to remember, concentrate, or recall language is encumbered.

Keep these factors in mind when you're questioning your own ability to explain yourself, to make yourself clear to your partner. And vice versa—when you can't make sense of what your spouse or partner is trying to tell you, ask yourself, "What's going on here? Is there something else in the background that is making this experience upsetting, frustrating, infuriating, and depressing?" You especially will think along these lines if the two of you have enjoyed an effective and fluid form of communication earlier in your lives together—because you will long for it.

What about medication? How does it affect communication? When individuals are taking the correct medication for their particular illness, they should be able to communicate better. If someone has a disorder of his or her thinking that makes the person ramble or lose goal direction, one of the major tranquilizers should help him or her to communicate more directly and clearly. For example, if someone has a delusional belief that he communicates with God through a microchip in his brain, his wife will find this strange and worrisome. With medication, this idea should end, and he will realize that he has been ill. If someone is severely depressed, his thoughts will be sluggish, hard to put into sentences, and despairing. He will be able to communicate much more adequately with his wife when he is taking an antidepressant medication. If a woman is in a state of manic excitement, she will not be able to communicate well with her husband and will likely be irritable, inappropriately happy, talking too fast, and jumping from one topic to the next. However, once she is stabilized on lithium (or some other mood regulator) the couple will find their marital communication much improved.

These are examples of when medication improves communication. But what about situations in which medication impairs communication? This certainly occurs when someone is overmedicated, that is, taking too many medications that affect the central nervous system or taking too high a dose. It is like being stoned, drugged, or drunk. Another adverse effect on communication is the result of disinhibition—medication causes the individual to lose his or her defenses or reservations so that what is said is too revealing or hurtful to the spouse. This can occur with some of the minor tranquilizers like diazepam (Valium) and lorazepam (Ativan) or sedatives like phenobarbital (Luminal) or secobarbital (Seconal). Another adverse communication effect of medication occurs when the drug actually affects the person's ability to speak, to form words and sentences clearly so that the spouse can understand. This can occur with the major tranquilizers like haloperidol (Haldol) or chlorpromazine (Thorazine), along with other side effects that can be relieved by lowering the dose, adding another medication to treat side effects, or trying another type of tranquilizer.

Before moving on to discuss specific psychiatric illnesses and their relationship to marriage, let me mention an often-observed and interesting point. There has been some research concluding that marriage works better for men than for women, that men are actually protected by marriage, whereas marriage can be psychologically unhealthy for women. Married men have less depression than single or divorced men, whereas married women, especially women with small kids and who do not do paid work outside the home, have the highest rates of depression. Married women with children are at risk of losing self-esteem and financial independence and at risk for battering and sexual assault by their husbands. They visit their physicians with various concerns much more often than married men. On the other hand, divorced men are prone to major medical illnesses such as heart attack, high blood pressure, stroke, and certain cancers and to psychiatric illnesses such as major depression, suicide, excessive drinking and other drug use, criminal acts, and death by accidents. Divorced men do not seem to fare well on their own or to want to be on their own very long—they remarry much faster than divorced women, and they remarry in greater numbers than women. In fact, many divorced women have absolutely no interest in marrying again, and they categorically state, "The last thing I want is another husband! I feel much happier and much healthier being on my own. Sure, I get lonely sometimes, but that's normal."

Questions

"My wife has had a severe depression before. Now she's depressed again. I hate it. I have to do the work she can't do because she's so sick. I'm exhausted, angry, and lonely. No one understands. I'm not sure I want to stay married. Am I just being selfish?"

Everything you're feeling is completely normal. It is very hard living with someone who is depressed, especially at the height of depression or when/if the person is having a recurrence. It's depressing and conjures up feelings of self-pity, anger, resentment, helplessness, and jealousy of others. "Why me? Why us?" are common questions. Depression is also probably the most common psychiatric illness that accompanies marital conflict, and, as I mentioned above, it can cause marriage trouble, be caused by marriage trouble, or both.

Some of the more common symptoms of depression are trouble concentrating, inability to listen for long, slow thinking, distorted or obsessively focused thinking, suspiciousness, decreased energy, decreased interest in doing things, less or no interest in sex, irritability, poor sleeping, decreased appetite or overeating, increased dependency, and self-absorption. All of these symptoms affect marriage, especially communication, connection, function, and intimacy.

Suggestions

Get in touch with the National Alliance for the Mentally Ill, the National Mental Health Association, or the National Depressive and Manic-Depressive Association. They are clearinghouses of information. Your community may have a local chapter of these organizations or its own mental health groups. You can also do a lot of reading in addition to attending a support meeting.

Ask your wife's permission to accompany her to her next appointment with her psychiatrist. Prepare a list of questions and concerns that you can ask her doctor. Perhaps you can also determine with your wife and her psychiatrist how much of a role your marriage plays in her depression. If it's significant, ask the psychiatrist about marital therapy for the two of you, in addition to the individual treatment your wife is receiving. Don't be afraid to raise the question of a second opinion by another psychiatrist if you think it would help.

Try to remember how your marriage was before the depression began. Was it quite strong then but is it less so now? Is there a strong biological element to the depression? That is, does your wife become depressed with minimal stress in her overall life circumstances? If this is so, then it is less likely that marital strain is a problem contributing to her illness.

Are you prone to depression yourself? You may be depressed even if you've never been diagnosed with it before. Read up on depression and see what you find.

You and your wife may benefit from viewing *The Storm Within*, a videotape on depression produced by the American Psychiatric Association. It's excellent and should be available in your community for rental.

Don't forget that mourning is part of your distress about the return of your wife's depression. You are grieving what you once had or hoped to have in your marriage. There is a longing and a nostalgia for that. By obtaining more information about your wife's depression, you can come to better terms with this loss, especially if your wife's psychiatrist feels particularly hopeful about her prognosis.

"I suffer from panic attacks. I don't think my wife understands. She's pretty unsupportive. It's ruining our marriage."

I imagine that it would help your situation if your wife could talk to your doctor or if she would read something about panic disorder. There is also a videotape produced by the American Psychiatric Association titled *Panic Prison* that you and your wife should view together. This will explain clearly your disorder and the various types of treatments that can help.

Are you sure you're having panic attacks? Review these symptoms of panic disorder—bursts of severe upset or discomfort that last for at least a few minutes during which

- You sweat
- Your heart pounds or speeds up
- You shake
- You feel short of breath or feel like you're choking
- You have pain or discomfort in your chest
- You feel like you're going to vomit
- You feel like you're going to faint or at least feel dizzy
- You feel like things seem unreal or you feel detached from your own body
- You fear you're going crazy or dying
- You feel numb or tingling
- You feel chilled or flushed

Be certain that your physical health is good and that these symptoms aren't due to a medication or excessive drinking or drug taking on your part. If you are taking medication for panic disorder, that needs to be explained to your wife as well. She may be concerned about your use of medication, how much you take, if it's habit forming or addictive, side effects, and so forth. She may also wonder if there are any nondrug treatments that might work for you such as hypnosis, relaxation exercises, stress reduction techniques, yoga, meditation, avoiding caffeine, or exercising more.

What is most important is that both you and your wife understand that panic disorder is a psychiatric condition that is terrifying, very real, and painful. It is not a sign of weakness. It is fully treatable, and it shouldn't have to ruin your marriage. If it seems to be, even after your wife has more information on panic disorder, go to a marriage therapist in case there are other issues affecting your relationship that aren't being recognized or addressed.

"My wife is agoraphobic. She won't go anywhere. What kind of marriage is this? I'm going crazy living like this. Any suggestions?"

I suggest that you try to get as much help as you can. Call your local mental health agency about reading materials, support groups, videos, public forums, and other forms of information. The American Psychiatric Association Division of Public Affairs has information on this subject. See if your community has a branch of SECURE, a support group for agoraphobic individuals and their families. Ask your wife's permission to accompany her to an appointment with her therapist or to see her therapist alone. Bring in a list of your questions and ask if you can help in any way. Don't make any decisions about leaving your marriage until you and your wife have had at least one attempt at marital therapy to see if there are ways of improving your marriage despite her agoraphobia.

"My husband has bipolar illness. Whenever he goes manic, our marriage dies a little death. I know he's got a mental illness but it's so hard sometimes for me to accept this."

You are not alone. Living with someone who has the dramatic mood changes that can occur with bipolar illness is very difficult. Manic symptoms can really affect marital harmony and marital stability. You can see how his illness affects your marriage because he is not the same—he is unable to function. You can't count on him as a husband at these times. Not only do you have to try to hold up his end of things, but you also have to worry about him at the same time. He may deny that he is ill, so he argues and fights with you, casting you into the role of police officer or parent, when all you want to be is his wife and lover.

Sadness is very common in marriages in which one or both individuals have bipolar illness. There is a wistfulness for what once was, a time of marital function and cooperation, of growing and planning together, of doing things together, of being parents (perhaps), of being able to communicate about things, of good health. Lithium, and other mood stabilizers, may affect sexual interest and function. There can also be a dashing of hope and promise, of what you had both projected would be your future together as a couple. So there is remorse and fear of the prognosis. Is he always going to be like this? Will we make it as a couple? And there may be anger. Why me? Why him? Why us?

Never forget your humanness. In other words, no matter how much you understand bipolar illness and that your husband is *ill* (not *bad)* when he's manic or severely depressed, it's still very hard to accept. Or it may be possible to be compassionate and patient one moment but impossible the next. You have your own personal needs and limitations—you are human.

You may feel that there are elements to your husband's disorder over which he has no control and that you can accept more than others. But if he's drinking excessively or taking street drugs, then you may be furious at him. Or if he stops taking his lithium and becomes manic or misses his doctor's appointments and doesn't cooperate with medical management of his condition, then you may get fed up. This can lead to marital erosion, division, and possible separation. If this is happening, marital therapy may help. His reasons for noncooperation may be complex, but one of them might be that he hasn't fully accepted his illness yet, so he thinks he's fine without medicine.

Perhaps you could join a support group for families with bipolar illness. Check to see if there is a chapter of the National Alliance for the Mentally Ill or the National Depressive and Manic-Depressive Association in your community. Meeting with other people who themselves have bipolar illness or who know the disease intimately because a family member has it can be reassuring. And you won't feel so alone with your feelings.

"My wife is being treated for an eating disorder. We have a lot of fights over food. Her doctor tells me to stay out of it. I can't. I can't let her starve herself to death."

As you probably know by now, an eating disorder can range from quite mild to very severe. The two basic eating disorders are anorexia nervosa and bulimia nervosa, and both can have a profound effect on the family. It sounds as though your wife suffers from anorexia and may be losing too much weight.

Your anxiety about your wife is perfectly understandable. Your inability to ignore her eating problems may be caused by many different factors. If she is in no immediate danger, you will have to step back and let her work with her doctor and nutritionist about her weight. If you don't "let go," it introduces too much control into your relationship; it casts you into a parental role, and this kind of role is never healthy in marriage. Her therapists are probably doing their best to teach her to be autonomous and in control of her own life, even if she is quite self-destructive. But if your wife's health is precarious and she really is very ill and unable to fully appreciate how life-threatening her behavior is, then you will have to intervene with vigor. Her doctor should understand that you are not being controlling or overreacting, you are merely being humane and sensible. I suggest that you talk to your wife's doctor again, just in case there has been some misunderstanding between the two of you.

One caution: look closely at yourself and try to determine whether you are "codependent." Are you reinforcing your wife's problem by inadvertently doing things that make it worse? Examples might be commenting that she's too fat or too thin; telling her that she shouldn't be eating this or that; being so controlling in another area of your marriage that she, in part, uses food to get back at you; refusing to see that maybe, because of your own insecurities, you "need" her to be sick so that you can feel strong; and refusing to see that maybe you have a need to be a caretaker and you need someone to look after to make you feel good about yourself. If you come from a background in which one or both of your parents were alcoholic or drug dependent, you might very well be codependent. Try reading one or more of the many books on codependency that are available.

I suggest that you consider one of several options. You might benefit from therapy yourself. It is difficult to live with someone with an eating disorder and hard to understand the illness. Could you benefit from a support group? A group for family members who have a loved one with some kind of medical or psychiatric problem is one possibility. Even better would be a support group for husbands of women with eating disorders. See if there is one in your community. If not, give some thought to starting a discussion group yourself.

Another option is marital therapy. You and your wife may indeed benefit from seeing someone together about your marriage. There may be some other problems that need addressing (e.g., money, your family, her family, your job), and they may be connected in some ways that you can't see with your wife's eating disorder. But you can probably both use a third party to help discuss matters that are hard to discuss at home.

You may want to discuss the lying and deception that often ac-companicompany eating disorders, or your mistrust of your wife, or manipula-tion, or the fear that your wife might commit suicide. She may want to discuss how much she feels you try to control her, the fears she has that you might abandon her, or her need to become more in touch with her feelings and to become more mature and more responsible for her actions.

You both might want to discuss how this problem has affected your marriage—the sadness you feel, the exhaustion and dispiritedness you both feel about its chronicity, the loss of the good times that you used to have together, the destruction of your intimacy as a couple, the threat to your sexual relationship—the growing fear, or sense, that your marriage might end.

SEVEN

The Role of Children in Marital Disharmony

The majority of people who marry want to have children at some point in their lives together. Childbearing and child rearing are perhaps the most profound periods in the lives of adults. In effect, people are changed forever when they become parents. Some individuals state that they can barely remember their lives *before* children.

Childbirth is a happy and exciting event for most couples. It is a time of deepening intimacy and individual maturation as this new phase of the marital life cycle is experienced. Usually this phase is reinforced by the excitement of the couple's parents, other extended family, friends, and work colleagues, who shower the parents and the child with gifts. Religious and cultural rituals also serve to honor and welcome the new baby into the world.

For many couples, however, things are not as blissful as they expected or were led to believe. Sometimes the stress may become overwhelming if they are struggling with severe marital conflict, immaturity, poverty, unemployment, physical illness, psychiatric illness, inadequate health care, and isolation from family support and friends. The stressors may be different for women and men.

Issues for Women

Many other books have described the phenomenal physiological and psychological impact of pregnancy, labor, delivery, and motherhood on women. Fatigue is the hallmark of the first several months of the new mother's life. If she is breast-feeding, this is especially so because she cannot share some of the feedings with her husband, and she has to sleep whenever she can.

Today, many women must adapt not only to becoming mothers but also to being somewhat isolated. Their role in the workplace has changed, and they may have less company of associates and friends. The length of this period depends on whether this is merely a maternity leave with return to work in a defined period or whether the woman plans to be a full-time mother and homemaker indefinitely. Given the insecurity of many marriages today, women may also feel threatened by the enforced financial dependency on their husbands until they resume working outside the home. Money equals power in contemporary society. Earning your own money, even if the sum is nominal, gives you strength and independence.

For those mothers who have returned to their jobs or careers, balancing work with their responsibilities in the home is a challenge. Arranging reliable child care via day care, in-home baby-sitters, live-in or live-out nannies, or a family member is central to peace of mind. Even then, many mothers feel torn and sometimes guilty as well. A supportive and helpful husband can make the difference between success or failure, order or chaos, joy or sorrow.

There are numerous physical changes that new mothers experience. Feelings of despondency and unhappiness, including crying, aren't uncommon during the postpartum period. (This is not the same as postpartum depression, which is a serious psychiatric/medical illness.) Accepting the changes in one's body requires time, explanation, and reassurance. I am referring here to changes in breasts and nipples, more weight than before the pregnancy began, stretch marks, lax vaginal muscles, widening of the hips, and, with cesarean section, an abdominal scar. There may also be a temporary problem with intermittent incontinence of urine and/or hemorrhoids from the pregnancy and the labor and delivery. All of these changes, plus lack of sleep, can affect one's interest in relationships and sex or one's pleasure in sex.

Coping with other children plus the new baby also represents a challenge—especially balancing everyone's needs and anticipating the older child's acceptance of his or her new sibling. Trying to decide when or whether to have more children is also a theme in most marriages for the first 2 to 3 years after a baby's birth. This includes talking about and deciding on a safe, effective means of birth control and, for many couples, discussing a sterilization procedure (vasectomy or tubal ligation) if the decision is not to have more children.

Issues for Men

Fathers have become much more directly involved with the care of their children over the past generation. We now have a better understanding of their psychological and emotional struggles as parents. It has been said that human fatherhood is fundamentally a social invention and that there are fewer cultural guidelines for fathers than for mothers. Contemporary fathers, and their wives, know this very well; many state that their own fathers were not role models because they were out of the home working and not that involved in day-to-day direct caregiving. So many of today's dads are really trailblazers in the home as they work at becoming fathers who are intimately involved in their children's lives.

When their wives become pregnant, many men do not realize that they are also evolving psychologically in preparing for fatherhood. Other men may be very aware; they begin to worry that everything may not go smoothly, that they may not be able to afford the child, that they may not be a good father, that they may not be happy whether it's a boy or a girl. Some men also feel shut out or excluded by their wives, who get all the attention. And if their wives are having difficult pregnancies, then they feel even more shut out emotionally and sexually. Their thoughts may turn to their childhood as they recollect memories of their own fathers. Prenatal classes serve many purposes, but one of the most important is as a vehicle for getting expectant fathers more involved with the pregnancy.

Some men have a very difficult time during the pregnancy or during the first year of their baby's life. More specifically, they may develop a psychiatric illness like an anxiety or panic disorder or a clinical depression. These illnesses are more common in men if they are genetically predisposed to develop them. Some men begin to drink as a way of dealing with stress and as a way of avoiding dealing with marital matters. This often leads to arguing and fighting, or physical violence, which may be completely out of character for the man.

Some men have affairs at this time. Affairs may work over the short term to help men feel loved, understood, listened to, or regenerated sexually. But over the long term they usually only confuse matters more. And, of course, affairs are especially painful for wives who already feel disadvantaged with their pregnancy and weight gain or, if they are postpartum, with their changed and maternal lactating body.

Even when it's a joint decision to have a baby, some men act as if there is absolutely no change in their lives. They make no effort to plan and prepare the nursery or to shop for the baby, and when the baby is born, they do nothing or very little to help. They may resent

He Says . . .

"She spends too much money, especially on clothes."

When I hear a complaint like this, I have several thoughts and questions. How domineering a husband is this man? Is this his wife's way of having some control in the marriage? Whose money is it, anyway—his, hers, or theirs? Do clothes make her feel good about herself? Is new clothing a bit of a pick-me-up? How serious is this? Is she bored with her life? With her husband? Might she be a compulsive shopper? Is this a type of addiction? If so, does she herself feel that she's out of control? Or finally, is this woman quite self-centered and insensitive to her husband's very realistic worries about money?

giving up their freedom or independence, so they balk at being asked to help out at home. Sometimes they are simply immature and need to grow up and become more responsible. Sometimes, and this is worrisome, they are selfish and put themselves first in most matters. But some men are only irresponsible on the surface; underneath they feel very inept and anxious about holding the baby, feeding and bathing him or her, changing diapers, being alone with the child, and so forth. Further, they feel threatened by or jealous of their wives, who seem to be adapting to motherhood with ease and competence. When their wives try to teach them basic skills for caring for a baby, they may feel defensive about their own incompetence, or they feel belittled. They may regress and become quite childlike themselves, which their wives find infuriating and certainly not cute.

Competitive feelings toward one's child are normal and should be expected to some degree. So don't feel guilty if you wish you could breast-feed or be cooed at or snuggled like your new son or daughter. It takes a while for new parents to get used to sharing each other with the new baby, especially someone who is completely helpless and who demands and needs so much. Once this phase passes, most parents know that the original relationship, the marriage, needs to be revisited and revitalized and that it is unhealthy and damaging to expect a baby to meet all your needs.

Issues for Couples

If you have been together for at least 2 years and are both fairly mature, and if you have often discussed having a child and have come to an agreement together, then it is easier to adjust to the new reality of your marriage. Further, if you're blessed with a supportive and helpful family and some good friends, those factors help a lot too. If your pregnancy is unplanned, or wanted by only one of you, then it may be tougher. The key is communication. Try to talk out your hurts, disappointments, guilt, anxieties, or sadness. This takes a lot of time, patience, and guts, but it will serve you well over the long term. You need to build or rebuild trust and solidarity in your relationship.

Always try to remember that you are a work in progress. You don't become parents overnight—you must grow into the role. You have to accept that you will make mistakes, that you can't always find the answers in a book, that often you will just be doing your best with the natural ability and skills you have. If you're going through a bad phase, try to remember that you are also mourning—mourning a life you once had, a life without kids, a life without a partner. That former life may be idealized, but your fantasy is that you were happier then or that life was easier.

Now you have to "schedule" your lovemaking, perhaps for the first time in your lives together. You long for the old spontaneity! If you're nervous about suddenly getting pregnant again, say so and talk about it. Discuss contraception, or a better form of it, with your doctor so that you can feel more at ease in the bedroom. It's a tall enough order getting used to sex again during the postpartum period without having to worry about another pregnancy.

Once your baby is a few months old, give some thought to acquiring a good baby-sitter (if you don't have extended family nearby) so you can begin to have brief dates with each other. One or two hours in a neighborhood coffee shop or restaurant can feel like heaven when you haven't been out alone together in months. The frequency and length of time away from your baby can be stepped up gradually as everyone acclimates and as your budget allows. And it is a good habit to get into. You are making an important statement to each other: "I care enough about you to want to be alone with you for a few hours."

When Marital Distress Affects Children

Most couples who are having marital troubles worry about the well-being of their children. Parental anxiety is reflected in the following questions and comments I hear from parents:

- "Are they picking up our tension? Our unhappiness? Did they hear us fighting last night?"

- "This is certainly not a healthy atmosphere in which to grow up. What kind of role models are we for when they grow up and marry?"
- "I feel so guilty; they don't deserve this unhappy home. I wonder if they're afraid that we might separate. Rebecca's wetting the bed, Sam's picking fights with everyone at school."
- "Do they really believe my explanation that Daddy's sleeping down in the basement because his snoring keeps me awake?"
- "When David says to us 'please don't fight again,' I just want to die."

What You Can Do

Accept the fact that your children probably know that something is amiss. This is true even if you have tried your best never to argue in their presence or within earshot or to cover up inner feelings of anger, fear, or sorrow. There may be no open tension in your home, but they may sense a vague or ill-defined change in the emotional atmosphere, that you are cooler to each other, or that you are leading increasingly separate lives.

Don't dwell on your guilty feelings in a passive, immobile way. This will only aggravate your state of unease and make you feel worse, more worried, more disappointed in yourself, and more angry at your spouse. Do something active about your situation; you'll feel a lot better for it.

Sit down with your child or children so you can explain a bit of what's going on. It's best if the two of you can do this together because *both* of you are parents. However, it is not always possible to talk with your kids together: you may not be speaking to each other; you may not be able to discuss anything, including telling the kids, without disagreeing; you may be the only one at home when you notice your kids are upset and you feel obliged to explain or to answer questions honestly; only one of you may value the importance of direct communication with your children in that your spouse minimizes the children's upset or takes a denying or protective stance toward the children; or you or your spouse may be engaged in an alliance with your children against the other parent so speaking to the children alone reinforces this.

When at all possible talk to the kids together. Accept that it's not easy to do this. Tell your children that the two of you are going through a very difficult time in your marriage. Obviously your language will need to be tailored to the age and psychological sophistication of your kids. "This is why I've been crying so much," "This is why we've been yelling so much at each other," and "This is why I've been so grumpy with you kids" are common explanatory statements. A statement like "We're trying our best to work things out" helps. And if you've sought marital therapy, tell the kids, "We're going to see a doctor (or counselor) about our marriage, just like I take you to a doctor when you're sick. We hope that this will help," and "Do you have any questions?"

The children may ask, "Are you going to get a divorce?" Be as clear and definite as possible. If divorce is unlikely, say "No, we're pretty sure we can work this out with some help and more time passing." If things don't look very optimistic, say "We hope not; that's why we're going to see someone to help us. We still love each other a lot, even though it might not seem that way to you. We want to try to stay together as a family." If you are going to be living apart, you can still say "No" to the question about divorce and add "We are going to separate, though, for a while and see how things go. If things get feeling good again, then we will get back together." You may want to explain in more detail the mechanics of your impending separation, as you know them at that point.

Reassure your children.   "This is not your fault that we're so unhappy. We're unhappy because of our own problems with each other. We both love you very much." Because children naturally tend to blame themselves for their parents' separation, you need to state these words aloud. And you may need to tell them more than once. The thought of separation can be very frightening to them so you must give them information and be there to answer their questions: "Is Daddy going to move out? Is he moving far away? Will he still visit us? Can we stay at his new house sometime? Do we have to move houses? Will you be OK, Mommy?" This is a time of major transition for all of you.

If your children are having symptoms (headaches, tummyaches, bedwetting, temper tantrums, trouble sleeping) that you think might be related to the problems at home, or if you're simply worried, take them to your family physician or pediatrician so they can be assessed. He or she may want to rule out any possible organic reasons for the symptoms. If there are none, the doctor may want to refer them to a child psychiatrist, child psychologist, or child treatment center for more study and treatment.

Speak to your day-care personnel, nanny, and teachers about your children and your observations, and give them a bit of information about the marital strain at home. This alerts them to any changes they see and enables them to be more observant, kind, supportive, patient, and comforting.

When Children Cause, Precipitate, or Aggravate Marital Distress

I am not using the word *cause* here in a blaming or pejorative sense. I am referring to those situations in families wherein the problems of a child have a tremendous impact on each of the parents, which then affects marital harmony. Most parents have had at least transient marital discord because they're worrying about a child or because they can't agree on the child's problem or its management.

You may have a child who has been "vulnerable" since birth—vulnerable to various physical and psychological events if he or she was born with cerebral palsy, congenital heart disease, cystic fibrosis, or asthma. Learning disabilities, with or without hyperactivity, are another kind of stressor. Vulnerable children usually require more professional attention as well as parental attention. This can be tiring and emotionally draining, especially if your child has a problem that is not easily diagnosed or not readily treatable. Other members of the family may feel shortchanged by one or both adults because of this child's special needs.

Your child may have a primary childhood psychiatric illness such as mental retardation, autism, a feeding or eating disorder, Tourette's syndrome, bedwetting, or fecal soiling. These are all challenging and often frightening and confusing disorders and can strain the best of marriages. And because of the stigma associated with many psychiatric illnesses, the pressure on your marriage may be worsened.

Your child may be passing through a normal developmental phase, a phase that is notoriously difficult for parents. One example is the so-called terrible twos. Another is a preadolescent and prepubertal stage in both boys and girls. And many phases of adolescence may be hard for the child and his or her parents. Children vary tremendously in how they cope with all of the hormonal and psychological changes of adolescence, for example, accepting the changes in their bodies, having an upsurge of strong sexual feelings, developing affectionate feelings (their first boyfriend or girlfriend), balancing time with their friends with time for school, competing in sports, and having their first job.

One parent may feel more aligned with the child and think that the other parent is being excessively strict, rigid, cruel, or indulgent. This polarization can cause demoralization in the marriage, particularly if exacerbated by a child who tends to play one parent against the other. I have seen parents conclude, inappropriately, that their marriage is dysfunctional when it actually isn't. The issues resolve when the couple doesn't have to worry so much about the children or once the children have grown and are no longer living at home.

Stepfamilies

What about blended or stepfamilies? This is one of the most common situations in which a child seems to precipitate marital strain. The source is usually ambiguity concerning the role of stepfamily members and in expectations of behavior and discipline. Quite simply, no one knows how to act or how to respond to a problem. It is extremely difficult for a stepfather or stepmother who has never had children to step into the role of parent, even when asked. Stepparents who have their own biological children find parenting a bit easier because they've had some experience.

It is not uncommon for the biological parents to experience a divided loyalty to their child and to their spouse. They try to please both and in this process often feel that they strike out. They can't please anyone, and they're always caught in the middle, upsetting one or the other. However, as painful as this is, it may be the healthiest of positions to be in. For if they are always siding with their child, their spouse feels invalidated and estranged, and there is real danger of the marriage ending (many second marriages end precisely for this reason). And if they are always siding with their spouse, their child (who was present *before* this marriage) feels betrayed, usurped, and alienated. This can cause depression, school failure, and acting-out behavior in kids.

It is true that after going through a divorce some biological parents have an especially strong, and not always healthy, bond with their child. This usually began years earlier, when it became evident that the original marriage wasn't working. The parent began to get too many needs met by the child, needs that weren't being met by the spouse. This tight bond was solidified during the divorcing period and during the period of adjusting to living on their own. "It's us against the world" is the modus operandi. This is more commonly mother and child, but not always—many fathers have a very tight binding relationship with their child, even when they are the noncustodial parent.

> ## She Says . . .
>
> **"He's obsessed with money and works long days and even some weekends. I don't care about material things anymore. I just feel empty."**
>
> One of my first questions is "Why is he obsessed with money?" Has he come from a financially insecure background? Is he trying to maintain a certain standard of living? Does money regulate his self-esteem to some degree?
>
> There are different ways of defining masculinity in North America: good looks, physical strength, athletic ability, intelligence, education, sexual prowess, endurance for hard work, occupation, and wealth, to name a few. All men will have more or less attachment to one or more of these because these are some of the things that define their maleness, their inner sense of themselves as men, their subjective sense of masculinity. These are also the things by which many men are judged by others (especially other men) as to how closely they attain ideal masculinity. It's certainly possible that your husband is trying to realize one of these objectives.

Depending on how painful the divorce is, or how difficult the adjustment is to separation, there may be a fair amount of guilt driving either, or both, of the parents. This gives the parent-child relationship a particular cast that is usually obvious to the stepparent. Here's an example:

Paula and Tim

Paula and Tim came to see me for what they called "separation therapy." They told me that they had tried everything to make their marriage work—and it all failed. They then decided, somewhat intellectually (they hid their feelings from each other), that they should separate. But this was hard because they each dreaded going through another divorce, and they didn't want to feel like "two-time losers."

Here's what I learned about their marriage. They had been married for only 2 years but had lived together for 2 years before that. Paula had a 10-year-old son, Mark, who had been a behavior problem for years. His problems, especially at school, had worsened in the past year. Tim characterized Mark as the source of their marital difficulty and the cause of their impending separation.

> I'm not just blaming Mark, even though I can hardly tolerate the little bugger; I blame Paula too. She lets him get away with murder. He's got her wrapped around his little finger; he cons her all the time. And she won't let me say a word. If I do, he tells me, "Go f____ yourself." Nice kid, huh, Doc? Or Paula steps in and yells at me for upsetting her precious baby. As you can see, I'm pretty burned up about all of this. We used to have a great relationship. Now it's the marriage from hell.

Paula agreed with most of what Tim said. However, she characterized Tim as being "too rough, authoritarian, and demeaning" toward Mark in his manner toward him. She admitted that she was defensive of Mark and that she's a "softy." She said that she felt terribly guilty as a mother and listed many reasons for this: she was very young and immature during her pregnancy and didn't really have much prenatal care; Mark was premature and was delayed in his milestones; she had a postpartum depression and felt she was "neglectful of Mark." Mark had a severe learning disability, and Paula wondered about his inheriting this from her. On a couple of occasions Mark's father had been violent toward him and she blamed herself for not leaving his father sooner. Now she felt guilty for putting Mark through yet another trauma, the loss of his relationship with Tim, which originally was not as bad as it had become since the marriage.

Therapy was very helpful for Paula and Tim, and they didn't separate. I saw them for only a few sessions, but this helped defuse the problem issues. I pointed out that Mark really was going through a very difficult time, on top of both a genetic and environmental predisposition to learning difficulties, and acting out antisocially. Mark began to attend a child psychiatry clinic, which was helpful both for him and for Tim and Paula. She was able to let go of much of her guilt and mobilize more energy for her marriage. She also became much better at setting limits with Mark. As Tim became more secure in his marriage, he was able to be more balanced in this relationship with Mark. He began to spend more time with Mark and to have some fun, rather than simply react angrily to Mark's unpleasant behaviors.

A Strain in the Second Marriage

Let me turn now to the situation in which the second marriage is already strained for its own unique or idiosyncratic reasons. What impact might this have on the stepchildren? This is difficult to sort out, often because everything may interact in a circular manner, so no specific cause is definitive. What I mean is this: If things are not going well in your marriage, this may cause you worry and sadness or irritability; this, in turn, may affect how you will be with your children or stepchildren. So they feel its impact, and this may cause them to behave in ways that suggest a threat to their equilibrium. They begin to act up or act out, which affects you, making you feel tense or guilty, which you then bring back to your marriage. Hence the vicious circle.

What is important here is that the children don't get blamed or scapegoated for your intrinsic marital troubles. This means that you and your wife, or husband, have to take an honest and courageous look at your relationship and try to determine which problems you two clearly own and in which ones the children may play a part. If it's still not clear after you consider this carefully, I suggest having a marriage assessment by a professional who can take an arm's-length look at the many issues that color your lives together.

If you decide to get some marital therapy, and many people in second or subsequent marriages do, make sure you tell your kids and stepkids that you're doing this. They will be greatly relieved and reassured. And if they haven't noticed any strain in your relationship, there isn't any harm in their knowing about what you're doing. It's largely a myth that telling kids about marital therapy might frighten them. It's actually excellent role modeling. From a very early age you are teaching them how important marriage is and that you value its health and preservation enough to get help. When they form their own adult relationships, they will likely embrace the idea of getting help, without feeling stigmatized or that they have failed in some way.

Issues Unique to Stepfamilies

Let me say a bit more about some of the differences between stepfamilies and conventional families. It helps to remember that each of you has experienced a loss from the earlier family that broke up and that there will be some scars from that. Also, each of your children has a parent from that family, and that relationship is extremely important, even if visitation might be irregular and strained. Your children came before your remarriage, and you and your spouse may not have had much time or opportunity to forge a strong couple relationship along with your involvement with the children. There may not be much sense of family cohesion or loyalty, at least at first.

If you and your spouse are blending two families, this can be very threatening and confusing for your kids. This is especially true if you will be moving to a new city or neighborhood, changing school districts, and leaving friends and family members. The kids may be sharing bedrooms in addition to sharing one-on-one time with you or your spouse. Almost everyone is experiencing some very strong emotion. Regular family meetings, once a week, can be extremely beneficial in giving everyone a voice or promoting the sense of family solidarity and teamwork. At first, it may be chaotic, and all of you may question the wisdom of your decisions. Most often, however, everyone shares the benefits of the stepfamily over the course of time. The Stepfamily Association of America (SAA)[1] has an excellent Educational Resources Program and many books for sale.

Points to Remember

- Pay attention to the health of your marriage and try to get some understanding as to how much your children contribute to marital harmony and disharmony.
- If problems with your marriage and children are not resolving, go for professional help.
- Even when worries about the kids are placing a strain on your marriage, the first treatment approach may be couples or marital therapy. This can help the two of you tackle the problem with children or stepchildren as a team or a collective so that you will feel a sense of mutual alliance.
- Things may then improve at home.
- Your child (or children) may need to be assessed by a child psychiatrist for his or her own individual and specific treatment. This may be a relief for you, after getting over the initial anxiety of introducing this to your son or daughter. If this progresses well, and you receive sufficient feedback and guidance from your child's therapist, your marriage may get back on track.
- Family therapy may be helpful in which all of you meet with the therapist to iron out the problems at home. Together you come up with solutions to the problems so that family function and solidarity returns, and people feel happy again. Your family doctor should be able to determine whether this kind of approach is best for you.

---

[1]Stepfamily Association of America, 215 Centennial Mall S, Suite 212, Lincoln, NE 68508. Telephone: (402) 477-STEP.

References

Erikson EH: Childhood and Society, 2nd Edition. New York, WW Norton, 1963

Myers MF: Marital upset after the baby. British Columbia Medical Journal 31:483–485, 1989

Visher E, Visher J: How to Win As a Stepfamily. New York, Brunner/Mazel, 1982

EIGHT

What About Separation and Divorce?

For most couples who separate, the decision has been a long time coming, and usually there has been a lot of discussion. And for most, this discussion has not involved the services of a trained professional. For some couples, a decision to separate is made hastily because of a painful and acute marital crisis. In these situations, the decision to separate has usually been made by only one partner. The partner who is "left" feels terrible—powerless, bereft, abandoned, and discarded. In some types of marital crisis, even the person who has initiated the separation and leaves may be very uncertain, ambivalent, and frightened, although it can certainly appear otherwise to the spouse and to family and friends. Indeed, some of these situations are so calamitous that they become, in essence, psychiatric emergencies, whereas certain other separations are rooted in existing psychiatric illness.

What do I mean by this? In human beings, separation can be a response to feeling threatened, extremely anxious, profoundly depressed, or disoriented and confused. As a marital therapist and psychiatrist, I have seen people leave each other under many different and sometimes extreme circumstances. Some examples are

- During a hypomanic or manic phase of bipolar disorder (manic-depressive illness)—or in response to a manic spouse
- Separation in an attempt to preserve one's own sense of well-being by leaving a severely depressed spouse
- Being in a delirious state and separating from one's spouse, or fleeing from a delirious spouse because of fear and misunderstanding
- Separating from a husband or wife who has become extremely paranoid and very threatening, with a wide range of irrational ideas and false beliefs
- Separating to preserve one's safety by running away from a violent or dangerous spouse
- Taking off in the middle of an acute stage of intoxication from alcohol or other drugs or in the midst of an alcoholic binge
- Walking away from a husband or wife who is alcoholic and who refuses to do anything about it
- Leaving home in the midst of a passionate and compelling extramarital affair
- Separating when someone is having a sexual identity crisis and is struggling with whether he or she is gay
- Separating during the early months or first year or two after the death of one's child
- Separating because of an accumulating number of personal and family stressors that have made living together overwhelmingly difficult

These are not stereotypical marital separations and certainly not the most common situations in which people find themselves deciding to live apart. At least in some of the above examples there is psychiatric illness in one or both of the partners that eclipses preexisting marital discord. The marital tension and demise that both partners feel are in large measure secondary to illness in one or both of them. These are marriages that may actually be quite healthy. They certainly cannot be adequately assessed until the psychiatric difficulty is diagnosed and treated.

If there is anything suggestive of the above situations in your marriage, I suggest that you seek the opinion and expertise of a psychiatrist or mental health professional. He or she can assist in many ways and with your assistance should be able to determine whether it is appropriate or necessary to separate. In fact, your therapist may even suggest that you put off separating if there is no danger (or possible danger) to you or your children. This will allow some time to pass so that each of you, and your relationship, can be thoroughly assessed. On the other hand, if there has been violence, or threats of violence (whether you see it or not), your psychiatrist or mental health professional will support or recommend an immediate separation. This may be temporary, but it will allow some time for cooling off, for safety, for some reflection, for some distance. There will not be hope for later communication

He Says, She Says . . .

He says: "I'm bored. I'm not sure if I love my wife anymore."

She says: "We hardly go out together as a couple anymore. When we do go out, he always wants to bring friends or family along."

I'm assuming that this man feels more than the usual boredom that all married people feel from time to time when they've been together a while and everything about the other is fairly familiar and predictable. In fact, he may have an unrealistic expectation of a wife: that she is supposed to be responsible for his personal boredom. Feeling boredom with life together as a couple is very different from a feeling of boredom with one's own life.

What might this husband say if his wife asked him about his apparent reluctance to go out alone with her? Perhaps he doesn't make the important distinction between being alone with his wife outside the home and being with her on a daily basis as part of the family. But if he really doesn't want to go out with her alone, she can't help but feel rejected, flawed, angry, and worried about their future together.

unless this finite period of separation occurs. As the ensuing days and weeks pass, each of you should feel less anxious, less angry, less confused, and less hurt. Then it will be easier to talk, both on your own and with the therapist's assistance. The possibility of reconciliation can be entertained only at this time and as a result of some efforts at communication.

Here is another type of situation. Let's say that your marriage is not in crisis but your relationship has been falling apart or unraveling for a long time. Both you and your spouse do not feel optimistic about turning things around, but you make a decision to consult a marital therapist to see if anything can be done. Perhaps you have already concluded that your marriage is over, but the two of you make a decision to call a marital therapist for help with separating. These situations are quite common and represent very solid reasons to consult a therapist, who can help with the separation. The therapist will make practical suggestions and answer questions but will also be available to comfort you, your spouse, and your family as you begin to go your separate ways.

Suppose you and your spouse are already in marital therapy, and separation becomes inevitable. It is important that neither of you sees separation as a failure of therapy. You haven't failed nor has your therapist. In fact, there's a lot that your therapist can do to continue to provide help and encouragement. So I strongly suggest that you both remain in treatment with that person for individual sessions as long as you feel is needed.

What do you do if you are about to separate and your therapist concludes that there's nothing more that he or she can do? There are some therapists who believe that their work with a couple ends when or if separation begins. You may not feel soothed, even if your therapist gives you names of other professionals that the two of you, or each of you, can see. If you've been seeing your therapist for quite a while, you will have established a deep relationship; you may not have the interest or energy to start working with somebody new, plus you already have enough on your plate with regard to your marriage and family. There are no easy answers to this dilemma. I suggest, though, that if you are currently in marital therapy, or if you are contemplating starting it soon, you discuss this matter immediately and find out about your therapist's policy.

What Does Separation Feel Like?

Most people do not know what to expect when they separate. It is new and unpredictable. There is a loss of one's base, perhaps a loss of a routine, and often much responsibility with children, work, or both. Most people who have gone through a separation and divorce have literally felt every possible emotion. When you physically separate, your feelings may come all at once or alternate rapidly from one extreme to another. And the feelings range from feeling horrible and lonely, to feeling sad and angry, to feeling scared stiff, to feeling relieved and ecstatic. If you've been thinking for a long time about separating, and if you and your spouse have been more or less leading separate lives before beginning to live apart, then you may not find living separately that difficult or that much of a change. On the other hand, if you have had virtually no warning about separation (even if there have been ongoing problems, you may never have thought that separation would occur, so that it hits with a thud), then you will find separation quite difficult. If you are completely opposed to it and have absolutely no control (or very little control) over your spouse's desire to separate, then living apart will likely feel terrible. Pay very close attention to your health because this kind of separation can be extremely traumatic to your physical and emotional well-being. If your friends extend a hand to you, by all means take it! And talk, talk, and talk some more.

Some people feel ashamed and that they've failed, as the following example illustrates:

Mr. D, an architect, came to see me several months after he left his wife. He was 53 years old and had been married for 23 years. While recounting the early weeks of his separation, he told me how self-conscious he had been during that time and how socially handicapped he had felt. The first time he went to the local supermarket to buy groceries, he found that his eyes were burning and that he couldn't see clearly. He was exquisitely aware of being on his own and of shopping for one. He was reluctant to look at the other shoppers in the store for fear that they might be staring at him. "I felt like a real loser and that everyone else who was shopping was either with someone or rushing home to have a meal with someone. All around me were sounds of families." Mr. D also recalled how difficult it was for him to go for walks on the beach, even though he had walked alone on the beach almost daily throughout his marriage. "I just couldn't do it, except at dusk when no one would be able to identify who I was. I just felt too conspicuous, too obvious."

Some people, healing quite nicely, find themselves backsliding when or if their former spouse meets someone else or gets married again. Here are the words of a 39-year-old woman:

> When my marriage ended, yes, I felt hurt and rejected, and sad. I expected from the beginning, though, that my husband would marry again. I thought I was over most of my pain until I learned that the woman he's marrying is 15 years younger than I am. That news has opened up old wounds for me. I feel even more discarded and useless than I did when we separated. Even though I'm outwardly a cynic and can be very sarcastic about men with younger women, I'm terribly hurt and lonely deep inside.

What About the Kids?

If you have children, you may want to see a family therapist who is experienced with working with the entire family or various members of the family, at times together and at times individually. But no matter whom you see, I suggest that you talk to a professional about what to explain to your children about separation, how to tell them, and when. The answers to these questions will vary depending on the ages of your children, the degree of openness in your family, how much they know or don't know about your marital difficulty, and what your separation arrangements are going to be. Your therapist may want to meet your children and talk with them after they have been told about the separation, or perhaps after the two of you have already separated. Depending on the ages of your kids, they may welcome the opportunity to meet with someone who has talked with many children in this type of situation. In fact, they may have questions and some fears that they don't want to mention to either of you. They may be attempting to spare you in some way, or they may be afraid of making things worse or of upsetting the two of you more than you may be already.

Another good reason for your children to meet with your therapist is that it gives him or her an opportunity to get some idea of how your kids are doing. If there is some concern on your therapist's part, then he or she can suggest a more complete assessment and possibly treatment by a child psychologist or child psychiatrist. Some communities have support groups for kids whose parents are divorcing, and these can be very helpful. And don't forget to let your child's teacher and the school counselor know about the separation. Most teachers appreciate knowing about changes occurring in the lives of their pupils. They can watch for any academic or behavioral changes in the classroom and, most important, provide that extra bit of support that is so comforting to children at a time like this.

Always remember that children, no matter what age, have feelings about their parents becoming separated. Because older adolescents and young adults are busy "growing up" and trying to become independent of their parents, there is a tendency to underestimate how they feel about their mom and dad living apart. They often act like it's no big deal, that their parents are free to do whatever they want, that they are too concerned with school, work, or their own friends to get upset. But they do react and often hide it or deny it. So try to encourage them to talk about their feelings, how they are adjusting to any new living arrangements, how they are coping with the ups and downs of each of you, and any worries they may have about money. They could have a lot of questions and they will hope that, despite the separation, their relationship with each of you will continue as before or may even get better. Be sure to reassure them of that, if you can.

Here's a challenge: Try to keep your personal feelings of hurt and rage at your spouse separate (as best as you can) from the needs and rights of your children to see their father or mother. It is very hard not to be punishing and vengeful by restricting your spouse's access to the kids or by undermining the visitation arrangement. But it is possible to tolerate if not succeed at this. One woman's words say it all: "I hate his guts and half the time wish he was dead. But he has every right to see the children, and they have every right to see him. I have to stand back and let their relationship continue."

What About Legal Counsel?

I suggest that you discuss the pros and cons of divorce mediation with your therapist in addition to the more traditional and conventional adversarial approach of divorce lawyers, who act solely for the individual. Mediation is purported to be much less expensive in the long run than paying two separate lawyers, but few separating couples feel confident and comfortable with the mediation process. In fact, many are in such pain that it is impossible for them to begin to consider sitting down together and working on an agreement with a mediator.

You may have many questions about joint custody, sole custody, and the implications of the various custody arrangements for you, for your spouse, and for your children. This is an important subject, and I therefore recommend that you have expert counsel by one or more professionals on these matters. It may also help to have the expertise of a child psychiatrist/psychologist, who may have something to say about the ages of your children and the stages of their development (and the relevance of this to a particular custody arrangement).

Extramarital Involvement

Like many people who are about to separate, you may already be involved with someone else. It is important to discuss this with your therapist because this makes your situation more complicated. It is especially more difficult for your children and complicated for your spouse. There will be anger and hurt associated with visitation, especially when it includes the third party. Do not just go ahead and introduce your new companion to your children. Discuss this with your therapist, who should be able to help you with your questions. Is there a good time, or an appropriate time, to have your children meet your boyfriend or girlfriend? Are your children ready? How might this affect your continuing coparenting relationship with your estranged husband or wife? Your therapist may even want to schedule a visit with you and your spouse together so that this situation can be discussed openly and frankly, because it may be very contentious. With your therapist acting as a go-between, the two of you may be able to reach some compromise and resolution of the strong feelings surrounding the introduction of this third person to the children.

If you are not involved with someone else but your spouse is, I urge you to be very assertive and forthright about your feelings regarding this person meeting your children. It is completely normal to feel protective and territorial about your children. It is also very normal to feel furious at your spouse for being involved with someone new or to be quite devastated about that relationship. Those feelings should soften and diminish as time passes. The old adage that time is the best healer is especially true—adjustment to your marriage ending and separation beginning does get easier as time goes on.

What About a Trial Separation?

Few couples separate knowing for certain that they will divorce. Some couples may contact a lawyer and begin divorce proceedings either before they separate or shortly thereafter, but these couples tend to be in the minority.

Almost every separation is a trial separation, although most are not given that designation. I say this because very few people know for certain that when they separate they will never reconcile at some point down the road. There are shreds of doubt and confusion in most people when they first begin living apart.

Having said that, what about a trial separation? Some couples do embark on their separation as a trial period—anywhere from 3 to 6 months—to see what becomes of their relationship while they are apart and how they fare living on their own. Every situation is unique. Some couples who separate more or less take it a week at a time. They may have some kind of loose arrangement about when they will see each other, if they will see each other, how much they will see each other, whether they are open to date others, and so forth. Some couples choose or decide right at the beginning not to see each other at all for a specific period (unless they have children, when of course they will see each other at transfer times and discuss matters regarding the children). These couples will try to keep their new lives as separate as possible, and each may have strong feelings of privacy. There may be an agreement to meet or to at least contact each other at the end of an agreed-upon time interval, say 1, 2, or 3 months. The idea is that each of them should have a clearer idea about how they feel about each other after some time has passed and whether they wish to consider or to actually work on a reconciliation.

There are other couples who are upset, angry, estranged, and not very hopeful about ever getting back together when they begin their separation. They may suspect that their separation will be permanent, but they are not certain. There remain some kind of ambivalence and often a deep and abiding commitment and caring about the other person. What they don't know at the outset is whether these feelings are healthy or even a valid reason for continuing the marriage, or reconciling at some point. In other words, they don't really see their separation as a trial separation, but yet they are not ready to see their marriage as completely over and they wait to proceed with divorce until several weeks or months have passed.

Some people are very cynical about the term *trial separation*. They see it as a cop-out, perhaps a euphemism, a gentle or nice term for divorce. I suppose that some individuals who are leaving a marriage and who feel quite guilty because they are hurting their partner may use the term *trial separation* to soften the blow. But most people who want a trial separation mean that quite literally; they need time, some distance, and some independence from their spouse because they are not really certain whether they want a divorce. Although many couples who begin a trial separation do not get back together and do go on to divorce eventually, there are others who reconcile and remain together happily. In fact, many couples will quite openly and boldly state that they would not be together today were it not for the trial separation that they had at an earlier time in their marriage. They may also make other statements that refer to the period of growth and understanding that they each accomplished by living apart for a while.

Let me make a comment concerning those who rankle at the term *trial separation*. These individuals, these husbands and wives, are generally feeling quite vulnerable, rejected, unloved, hurt, angry, and frightened. One of my patients, a 35-year-old accountant, said to his wife in my office when she brought up the subject of a trial separation:

Why don't you just hit me over the head with it? Be straight with me. Stop beating around the bush. Just say it. Tell me that you don't love me any more. That you hate my guts. That you're sorry that you ever married me. And that you want a divorce. You just want to get on with your life and forget that you ever knew me.

As you can see, these various separation options may not be easy to discuss. This is where your therapist can help the two of you talk about your wishes and your feelings. Even if you and your partner are able to discuss these things fairly easily at home with calmness, that may not be the feeling that you have inside. Each of you may feel a great deal of inner turmoil. And because some of your feelings are negative or critical of your spouse, individual visits with a therapist can be very helpful and more appropriate. It is best to say destructive and hurtful things to a therapist first as opposed to your spouse. This gives you an opportunity to get things off your chest without having to worry about causing more pain.

On the other hand, your therapist may want to meet with the two of you together from time to time, especially if there are concerns about the children, because meeting together is the best format in which to discuss family concerns. And if the two of you are having disagreements, fights, and hurt feelings about how much time you spend together, this may also be a good reason for sitting down with your therapist. He or she should be able to appreciate each of your positions and to determine whether a middle ground is appropriate or whether one position will have to be respected and honored more than the other.

Here are some examples of what I mean:

1. It is normal for each of you to feel a sense of privacy about your life once you have begun to live apart. However, one of you may feel this more strongly than the other. You may not want your estranged spouse to see your apartment, but she or he may feel quite hurt or rejected.

2. Your husband wants to "date" you. You have no interest in this at all. In fact, the only time you would want to see him or meet with him would be to discuss matters regarding the children. Ostensibly he accepts this but seems to come to the meetings with another agenda, for example, flowers, tickets to the theater, or questions about what is going on in your personal life.

3. You may want to get together from time to time "as a family." You say this because you see yourself and your husband or wife as rational and mature human beings who should be able to put feelings aside and have a nice family time for a few hours. Therefore, you feel annoyed or dispirited if your spouse says this is too hard or could be confusing for the children and may give them unrealistic or false hopes that the two of you might be reconciling.

4. You begin to have some concerns about your husband's morals—you don't like the idea of his new girlfriend staying overnight when he has the children with him for the weekend. You mention this to him and he becomes furious. He accuses you of being judgmental, a prude, jealous of his new life, controlling, interfering, and threatening him through the children (whom he argues he doesn't see enough of anyway). You may or may not be feeling any of what he has accused you of. What you are worried about is that the children have not had time to come to an acceptance that their mom and dad will not be getting back together and that Dad has clearly moved on and wants the children to come to know and accept the new person in his life.

The above are only a few examples of the many confusing, contentious, and difficult situations that can arise when people have separated and are living on their own. Most of these matters can be resolved quite nicely with the assistance of a therapist meeting with both parties, and I highly recommend it.

NINE

What You Can Do to Help Yourselves

There are very few couples who do not have doubts, worries, or concerns about their marriage from time to time. In general, people wonder if what they are experiencing is normal: "Are our problems common to most couples? What are the norms? Should we be worried?" They want to know what to look for, what they can use as a benchmark.

A small number of couples come for marital therapy when they first begin to experience marital distress. These are couples who have come from backgrounds in which there was terrible marital discord in the parents' lives, or one or both partners have been in a previous committed relationship or marriage that did not work. They know only too well the pain and anguish of marital unhappiness and divorce, and therefore they embrace help early to try to prevent or alleviate further distress.

Most couples who come for help have been distressed for a long time. Often there has been a cyclical pattern where the couple goes through a period of intense distress and unhappiness. At this point one or both of them often decide to get help. However, shortly after this decision is made, it is not uncommon for their situation to improve so that they lose their motivation to get help. For many couples these periods of distress return, and once they recognize the cyclical pattern, they will be more convinced that they need help. Couples who come for marital therapy very late in this process often make statements like "I wish we had come here 3 years ago (or 10 years ago)."

Pay Attention to the Warning Signs

So what should you look for as a warning sign of problems in your relationship? One of the best clues is the sense of something not being quite right within. This might mean that you are feeling tense or anxious; you have trouble sleeping; your appetite may be off; you find yourself irritable with family, friends, or co-workers; you are having angry outbursts; or you feel generally unhappy.

Physical symptoms can provide a clue. You notice that you are having headaches, an upset stomach, pain in your chest, dizziness, backache, or a change in your bowel habits. If you are someone with arthritis, asthma, diabetes, migraines, ulcers, or colitis, you may find that you are having more symptoms of these disorders than you have had in some time.

Another warning signal is related to your use of alcohol and other drugs. Are you drinking more than usual? Are you using recreational drugs? If you are already taking tranquilizers or painkillers, are you using more of these medications than you usually do?

Persistent thoughts about separation are another warning sign. Occasional or intermittent thoughts of separation are normal in all marriages, especially when people are arguing or are not feeling as close as usual. However, if you find yourself thinking about separation and divorce and are spending a lot of time planning what life would be like on your own, you may be in some type of problem-solving mode. These fantasies of separation and divorce can be comforting and can give you a sense of hope that there is a life after marriage. But if you also feel guilty about these thoughts, or terrified, it could mean that they are only one means of getting through the present. They may even be appropriate, if your marriage is not salvageable. With no other perspective, though, it is hard to know whether there is another solution besides separation. Use these thoughts as a springboard for going to marital therapy. This will assist you in finding out whether separation and divorce make sense for your situation.

What if you feel fine and have no psychological or physical symptoms at all, but your partner does? What if you feel perfectly happy in your marriage, but your partner is miserable? It is not unusual for only one member of a couple to feel that there is a marital problem. Also, it is not unusual for one partner to be upset about the marriage because his or her spouse is; that is, he or she was fine and thought the marriage was fine until the spouse began discussing it. The following is an example:

Bill and Sandy

When Bill and Sandy came for therapy, they had been married for 5 years and had two children ages 4 and 2. Bill thought their marriage was "wonderful" until he came home from work one Friday evening and found Sandy unconscious on the kitchen floor. Their children were hungry, unattended, and crying in an adjacent bedroom. Bill immediately called 911, and Sandy was taken to the emergency room. He learned later that she had taken an overdose of alcohol along with sleeping pills, which had been prescribed by her family physician. She was treated in the intensive care unit of their local hospital and was transferred to the psychiatric ward for a 3-week treatment of depression.

Bill was absolutely flabbergasted when he was told by Sandy's psychiatrist that she had been depressed for several months but had somehow hidden this from him. She had been living with a number of symptoms: poor appetite, trouble concentrating, insomnia, weeping spells, no energy, and excessive drinking. Bill hadn't noticed any of it. He was very busy with his own career and was out of town often on business. Because he was making good money, he could afford to have a "mother's helper" in the home to assist Sandy. He could not understand why she was unhappy.

There was much more to their situation. Sandy felt beleaguered by her responsibilities of being a mother to two young children, being a wife, and running their home single-handedly. She felt unhappy in the marriage because there was virtually no communication, their sexual life was programmed and unrewarding for her, and she had no sense that Bill respected and loved her. She was correct in many respects. Bill was certainly very busy and absorbed with his work, but subjectively he felt very committed to Sandy. He felt that he loved her and the children. The problem was his inability to communicate his feelings of love and tenderness, and this formed the basis of much of their marital therapy. They responded well, and within 3 months both were feeling that their marriage was much happier and certainly more functional. Bill cut back on his traveling and began to share more of the workload at home.

Some people have a marital problem but do not realize it until it is expressed by someone else in the family. An example is a situation in which your child develops symptoms such as frequent stomachaches, headaches, temper tantrums, bed-wetting, or aggressive behavior. You take him or her to the doctor, and the doctor cannot find anything physically wrong, nor can the doctor find any other stressors in your child's life like school, day care, or siblings. It is possible that your child is manifesting symptoms because he or she is picking up tension or problems in you. Any unhappiness that you might be feeling with each other is not being expressed directly between the two of you but is coming out in behaviors toward your child, such as excessive demands, rigid discipline, or a lack of structure and discipline. One word of warning: Do not jump to the conclusion that your child's symptoms are caused by your marriage without getting a professional opinion. It is quite possible that he or she is having symptoms for other reasons.

What I have talked about so far have been psychological and physical symptoms of distress in either you, your spouse, or your child. But what about marital symptoms in your relationship? What do I mean by marital symptoms? You might be bickering a lot, or nitpicking. You may find that you are not resolving arguments like you once did, and this is extremely exasperating. Issues may come up over and over again that, given your past pattern of communication with each other, should be resolved. You may find that your arguing is rapidly accelerating and you find yourself more insulting, hitting below the belt, swearing, threatening, or resorting to name-calling. If you are not finding this in yourself, perhaps you are noticing it in your spouse. It should worry each of you if you find yourselves prone to physical violence—pushing, slapping, or hitting—when this was not happening before.

If you are a person who is not particularly verbal and you find yourself even quieter and communicating even less, that is also concerning. It is especially serious if you are finding yourself withdrawing, retreating into silence, and withholding your feelings and affection from your spouse. If you are walled off, you may notice that you're unreceptive to affectionate gestures or sexual overtures from your spouse. Again, this should be a warning signal that something is not right. If you do find yourself accepting your spouse's affectionate or sexual overtures but in the process find yourself feeling cold, angry, or simply numb, consider this a warning signal as well. You should be able to tell if your communication with each other has changed drastically and if the way that you speak to each other is icy, clipped, or formal.

There are many other kinds of marital symptoms. Pay attention to the following signals and let them alert you to the need for help. Watch to see if you are actively avoiding your partner. If you find that you do not want to do anything together, pay attention. If you do not want to share or discuss anything with each other except mundane everyday happenings, that can mean that you have lost faith or trust in each other. If you never go out together as a couple alone but always want to socialize with others or with your family, it could mean that you are avoiding the intensity and possible intimacy of spending time together by yourselves. You may be avoiding it because it is too painful, tense, or dreary. Sometimes couples do not even remember what it feels like to go out together—it's been so long that they're afraid they will have nothing to say to each other. Fortunately they are sometimes pleasantly surprised when they actually have a good time.

Pay attention if you find that you are leading increasingly separate lives; that is, you rarely discuss matters with each other, you make plans without consulting each other, and you avoid spending one-on-one time together. If your way of life is becoming increasingly constricted and perhaps restricted only to your children, this can be serious. You should also note if the areas of overlap and shared activity and purpose in your marriage have become limited. If you find that your only reason for being together is the children, then you need to give that a lot of thought. A very important and poignant question is "Is my husband, is my wife, my best friend?"

Extramarital involvements are a common symptom or sign of a marriage in distress, as discussed in an earlier chapter. In fact, some individuals don't even realize they have a marital problem until they suddenly find themselves infatuated with someone else. It is only then that they recognize that things have not been as harmonious, close, or functional at home as they thought. Marital discord is not the only reason for an extramarital relationship, but it is one of the most common. It isn't unusual for someone to begin to reflect on his or her marriage only after meeting someone else.

The following is an example:

Henry and Lillian

When Henry and Lillian came to see me, they had been separated for 6 weeks after being married for 25 years. They separated when Henry announced that he was having a relationship with his secretary and had been for the previous 6 months. Understandably, Lillian was deeply hurt and outraged and asked Henry to leave that evening. He obliged, and they had been living separately since that time. However, they were having some contact with each other because of their three children ages 19, 17, and 15.

Henry said he was extremely confused about his situation. In many ways he felt deeply committed to and loving toward Lillian but he also admitted quite honestly that he was in love with his secretary. When I asked the two of them their reasons for coming to therapy as a couple, both of them said, almost simultaneously, that they were uncertain about whether their marriage was salvageable. Lillian was very clear, however, that she was not prepared to reconcile with her husband until his relationship with his secretary was finished, both romantically and professionally. Henry was not at a point where he could honor her wishes.

I made the decision to have individual visits with Henry and Lillian over the next few weeks. I saw Henry for psychotherapy so that both he and I could understand what was actually going on for him. He certainly had some frustrations about his marriage; he had more frustrations, though, about aging, about his advanced diabetes, his unhappiness in his firm, and his children, none of whom, he felt, was doing as well as he thought he or she should. I also found him to be moderately depressed. The therapy helped him develop a clearer sense of what he wanted in life. He began to feel that his relationship with his secretary was causing him tremendous anguish, and he could not continue to hurt both his wife and her. He made the decision to end the relationship with her, and he learned, much to his surprise, that she was relieved to end the relationship as well. They stopped seeing each other outside the office, and she gave her notice to leave and seek employment elsewhere.

After a few more weeks of reflection, and after taking a vacation abroad for a month to think, Henry returned with a goal of working on his marriage. Lillian was willing to explore this with him, and the two of them began to see each other on "dates." I also saw them for a few visits for reconciliation therapy, and they found it helpful to begin to talk about the many areas of concern that they shared. Their communication improved tremendously, and they found themselves feeling closer and more intimate than they had in 15 years. Henry decided to leave the firm in which he was a partner and to go out on his own. This was an important career decision for him, and this gave him a greater measure of personal happiness that extended into his behavior at home as both husband and father.

So far I have identified some of the more common personal and interpersonal symptoms that people experience in the face of marital discord. I have called them warning signals because they really are clues that something is not right. When we can identify why we are feeling the way we do, there is usually some relief.

So what can you do on your own as a couple to try to make things better? Or what can you do by yourself to try to improve things at home? Recognizing and accepting that there is a problem is the first step to a solution. But this is easier said than done. I find that there are at least two stages: 1) putting a label on that unpleasant feeling state or the negative interaction between the two of you, and 2) acknowledging that you play a part in the genesis or the reinforcement of that situation. This second stage is difficult because it is always easier to see the other person's contribution more clearly than our own. Or even worse, we feel that we have no part in it at all, that it is all generated by our spouse. Here is a rather simple example of what I mean:

Jim and Susan

One of the complaints that Jim and Susan brought to their therapy was that they had not made love in 6 months. They had a number of other stresses and problems in their marriage that were probably contributing to their sexual distancing from each other, but their communication on this subject was blocked. Both certainly acknowledged and recognized that their sexual frequency had diminished because they were used to making love about once or twice a week.

In one of their conjoint visits, I urged the two of them to try to talk about this, saying that I would offer assistance. Jim went first, and volunteered that he had not been feeling particularly interested in sex for some months because of the bankruptcy he was going through. He felt greatly preoccupied with financial matters, but more significantly, he also felt extremely humiliated by this process. To quote him, "My self-esteem has been terrible the past few months; I feel especially disappointed in myself as a man, and I think that this carries into the bedroom." I asked Jim to elaborate, and he mentioned that he was afraid to initiate lovemaking with Susan because he was afraid that he would have erection difficulties as a consequence of his very poor sense of his masculinity. When I asked Susan to respond to some of Jim's statements and concerns, she told him that she was aware that he was very worried about his bankruptcy, and she also felt that his self-esteem was probably greatly affected by this. He had made asides at times that gave clues to this, and he frequently made comments about how successful so many of their male friends were. Susan therefore elected not to suggest making love because she felt that this would pressure him and that he already had an enormous amount on his plate. When Jim heard this, he was greatly relieved and asked Susan, "You mean, you are still interested in me?" She responded with surprise and said, "Of course!" This was a telling moment in that session as both of them realized that they had been sitting on a lot of feelings about their sexual life together that had not been aired. They also became aware of the misunderstanding in that Jim had assumed Susan had lost her interest in sex and more specifically had lost interest in him. What Jim asked Susan to do was to take more initiative in their lovemaking and said that he would likely be much more responsive than he had been before, or than he appeared. This is, indeed, what happened, and the two of them were able to resume their healthy and loving sexual life together with ease.

Unfortunately, not all couples are able to talk about a recognized problem as easily as Jim and Susan were able to discuss their sex life together. Sometimes this is because only one of the partners perceives it as a problem, or they both perceive it as a problem but one person wants to deal with it and the other wants to ignore it. If their attempts to discuss it the first time around don't go well, it may be harder for one of them to bring it up a second time. And if that doesn't go well, it is unlikely that they will attempt again a third or fourth time.

How a problem is brought up in a relationship is critical. Much of this was explained earlier in the chapter on communication in marriage, but let me reiterate. If you bring up a concern to your husband or wife in a harsh or dogmatic way, or with any hint of accusation, you are virtually asking for and guaranteeing that your spouse will deny the concern or will attempt to argue a way out of it.

In marriage, it is common to have differences of opinion about problems, the nature of the problems, and even the duration of such. Therefore, one person may be very concerned and want to talk about it and work it out, whereas the other person does not see it that way. Most couples who come for marital therapy comment on this. Women tend to pay more attention to communication within marriage and are generally much more willing to go for professional help earlier than their husbands.

It's always easier to see one's partner's role in the problem or to totally blame one's partner. Sometimes this is caused by immaturity, sometimes it is due to lack of insight. Here are some common complaints or gripes that people have in marriage:

- "My husband drinks too much."
- "My husband has a violent temper."
- "My wife nags too much."
- "My husband only thinks about sex."
- "My wife has no interest in sex whatsoever."
- "My wife is too sensitive. She cries over everything."
- "My husband is extremely selfish. He thinks only of himself."

On the surface these complaints appear as psychological defects or shortcomings on the part of one or both partners. However, what is important to remember is that these are not absolutes, and there could very well be something that you are doing inadvertently or unconsciously to bring out these distasteful and unpleasant behaviors in your spouse. This is not easy to do because it means looking inward, but looking inward is one of the first steps on the path to marital recovery.

Improving Your Marriage on Your Own

You must begin to listen carefully to your partner. Work from the premise that his or her concerns are being aired in good faith, that he or she is trustworthy and is not trying to win some kind of imaginary battle or to put you down. As you can see, trust is fundamental because without it you cannot accept that your partner's complaint is sincere. Although trust is fundamental, and the bedrock of a healthy marriage, it is not always static in a relationship. It waxes and wanes. But it is very difficult to communicate openly, honestly, and with spirit when trust is weak or absent.

Defensiveness is a problem in marriage, although it is normal to feel defensive about many, if not most, of one's liabilities and insecurities. Feeling or acting defensive can be a normal reaction to threat, attack, or perceived criticism. All it means is that you are feeling anxious. The key is to accept that both you and your spouse will feel defensive when trying to communicate on many issues, especially the more sensitive ones. When we volunteer or admit that we are feeling defensive, it makes communication flow more easily. On the other hand, if we're criticized for being defensive, that just makes us feel worse or doubly defensive. For example, the statement "Stop getting so defensive!" tends to prompt the comeback of denial, "I'm not defensive!" I believe that this kind of interaction happens when people feel shamed by their spouse and respond quickly to ward off this painful emotion. My suggestion is that you keep working on this matter of defensiveness. It will diminish in time.

Gender Roles in Society

As we have seen, women tend to monitor the functional state of their marriage much more than do their husbands. However, increasing numbers of men are also concerned about the health and function of their marriage. Occasionally there is complete reversal where it is the man who is concerned about and committed to fine-tuning the marriage, and it is his wife who doesn't seem to be that interested or concerned about their communication, companionship, ability to solve problems, solidarity, affection, or sexuality.

The point is, *listen to your spouse.* Listen carefully to what he or she has to say about how you're doing as a couple. Pay attention when your spouse or partner wants to talk about how you do or do not communicate well with each other. Pay attention if your spouse or partner is concerned about your mood and your behavior. Pay attention if he or she wants to talk about articles in magazines on marriage or discuss a particular talk show or documentary about marriage. Understand that this is his or her effort to keep your marriage alive and healthy.

Many people cannot perceive the value of marital therapy. In fact, most men argue that they can solve things themselves; marital therapy is equated with failure. True, some issues are resolvable by paying extra attention. However, other conflicts are so complicated, contentious, or deeply rooted that they are impossible to resolve without help. It doesn't matter how intelligent, how well educated, how knowledgeable about psychological matters the two individuals are. Their efforts together just won't work.

Many women cannot understand the reluctance of men to go for professional help. Therefore, by the time a woman's husband agrees to go with her to see someone, she is exhausted and furious. She is exhausted because it has been so much work to get her husband to understand how unhappy she is or how disordered their relationship really is and furious because she has had to do all of this herself, and her husband's reticence or negativity does not make sense to her. It is not good enough to say "No, I won't go with you." Examine what you're feeling inside and share your reservations. Here are some of the more common reasons men give for not wanting therapy:

- "I'm a smart man, we're smart people, we can handle these problems ourselves."
- "Our problems really aren't that bad, are they?"
- "My parents went to a marital therapist for help—what a joke, they ended up divorcing."
- "What can a marital counselor do? Most of them are screwed up themselves."
- "We can't afford it."
- "Talking to a complete stranger about my problems really scares me—who wants to air their dirty laundry in public?"
- "I feel nervous going to see a counselor with you. I'm afraid that you and the counselor will pick on me or walk all over me. I can't hold my own as well as you can."
- "Why should we go to a counselor together? All you're going to do is complain about my drinking."
- "I went to see a marital therapist with my first wife. I never went back when he told me that I had a mother fixation. What a loser!"
- "It's embarrassing to go to see a shrink about your problems. If the guys at work knew that we were going to see someone, they'd really have a good laugh about that."

Accept That You Are Human

Like all married people, you are vulnerable to marital distress from time to time. Keep in mind that all marriages go through periods when they are much more stressed: for example, the first year after a child is born; the period in which you have one or more preschool children; when there is illness in the family; when one or both of you are unemployed; during the middle years of your life; when children leave, or don't leave; and around the time of retirement.

Many couples attribute their problems to overwork on both their parts. They acknowledge this as a sign that their marriage will not survive if they keep living like this. If it is possible for the two of them to cut back on their paid work and still meet their basic needs, many couples opt for this; in other words, they would rather have a simpler lifestyle and be happier. What they have realized is that they are paying a terrible price in terms of their companionship and intimacy by striving for a home or a bigger home in a better neighborhood, an exotic vacation, another car, and so forth. They start comparing themselves to their friends who *seem* to be able to keep up much better than they can and who always *seem* happily married.

The Influence of the Past

Pay attention to your personal background, how you grew up, and the family in which you were raised. The chances of your having a happy and successful marriage are much greater if you were raised in a home that was loving and secure. More specifically, if you have had role models as parents who felt a lot of love for each other and were committed to each other and to family, then you have probably learned much from them.

If your parents have divorced, you may be more prone to marital breakdown yourself. The reasons for this are far from clear, and it is certainly not a direct cause and effect. Not all children of divorced couples go on to get divorced themselves. In fact, most couples divorcing today have grown up in intact homes. If there is a history of violence in your family, then it is extremely important that you pay attention to this; violent tendencies tend to pass from generation to generation, and you are at greater risk for being violent with your spouse or children if you have been subject to this yourself growing up or if you witnessed violence in your parents' relationship. The same is true for certain psychiatric illnesses such as depression and drug dependency. If you, in turn, suffer from depression, alcoholism, or drug addiction, you are at greater risk for marital difficulty, separation, and divorce.

My purpose in mentioning the above factors is not to be depressing or alarming but to raise consciousness. When we have a better understanding of what makes us tick and how we have become who we are today, it is much easier for us to go through life with a sense of control, purpose, and optimism. This is not an absolute; it is merely a guiding principle.

The Work of Marriage

You must recognize and accept that all marriages require care, time, thought, patience, sacrifice, nurturing, and grooming. An enduring sense of humor is also a plus. These are not things that most of us think of in our everyday lives, but most people would agree that marriages do not function or thrive without at least some of these ingredients.

It is absolutely essential that you and your husband or wife make an effort to set aside time regularly to spend together as a couple. Most people find that once a week is a good time interval, but it should never be any less often than every 2 weeks. Setting aside time to be together gives you an opportunity for conversation, relaxation, romance, and possibly sex.

It is a worthwhile exercise to observe yourself and your spouse over the next few weeks to see whether the two of you do set aside time for togetherness. Pay attention if you observe that you "forget" to do it or if you feel you have been "far too busy" to get together. Note whether *you* might be actively avoiding setting the time aside, and observe whether you feel your spouse is actively avoiding making the time to spend with you.

Let me also make an additional suggestion with regard to setting aside time for each other as a couple. I recommend that you try to spend this time out on a date with each other. This, of course, will depend a lot on your budget and on the "busyness" of your lives. But herein lies a paradox—the busier you are in your respective and family lives, the more important it is to set aside time together as a couple. On the other hand, the busier you are, the harder it is to find time to spend together. If you (or your husband or wife) has a work schedule that demands your absence from the home for several days or weeks, then obviously you cannot spend time together, at least in person. You may be spending a fair amount of time together over the telephone, and that can be beneficial. If your lives are punctuated by frequent absences, it is important that you use the time that you do have together wisely.

Many couples find that they have their best conversations with each other outside the home. This is usually because the setting is different and it may even be more conducive to conversation. In other words, the setting could be pleasant like a restaurant, or a walk in a park, or the ambience of a coffee shop. But in addition to the actual setting in which you spend time together, you will not be subject to the interruptions that characterize the lives of busy people—the phone ringing, someone coming to the door, the children interrupting or awakening, the dirty laundry that needs to be washed, the grass that needs to be cut, and so on.

You must protect this time because if you don't, weeks will pass and you will notice that you haven't been out together. I suggest that you mark your "dates" on the calendar and don't allow other commitments to interfere. Some couples find that it is easier for them to set aside a particular evening of the week as their evening; other couple's schedules will not allow this, so they have to be flexible. What is important is that there be a date somewhere in that interval for the two of you.

Although these suggestions and efforts seem very logical, sensible, and rather simple, they are not always that easily instituted or sustained. In fact, many people find doing something like this quite foreign and completely impossible. They state that their lives are just too busy, especially if they have small children and many other commitments to their extended family, to friends, and to their community. I argue that it is especially important at this phase of one's life to set aside time for each other, because today people often have an overwhelming number of commitments. It is extremely common and very easy to lose sight of each other as friends, companions, and lovers in the midst of busyness. Many parents relate to each other as parents of their children as opposed to two adult individuals who had a relationship before they had children. If you have not grown up in a home with this kind of relationship primacy, it is all the more important to try this and to do it differently from your own parents.

I also suggest that you think honestly and seriously about the amount of busyness, especially overwork, in your daily life. Do you need to be as busy as you are? Are you avoiding responsibilities to your husband or wife by taking on so many commitments within your family or outside your family? Have you taken on a lot of these things because you find life with each other boring, depressing, empty, or riddled with tension? Is your overwork, then, a method of coping with an unhappy marriage? If the answer to any of these questions is "yes" or "possibly yes," I suggest that you talk to each other and see if there is some way you can begin to reconnect.

Couples as Friends

Try to meet and cultivate at least a few sets of close couple friends whom you can trust and with whom you can communicate. This takes time and work because it is not easy to find the right combination of four individuals liking, respecting, and enjoying each other. Most people find that they enjoy socializing with other couples, especially ones who are relatively close friends. One other benefit of being friendly with one or more couples is the opportunity to share common experiences. Therefore, other couples can be an invaluable source of comfort, support, and reassurance, especially during periods of marital distress.

Couples who are a bit more seasoned, a bit older, who have been together longer, or who have experienced and survived their own share of individual and marital troubles can provide a reassuring sense of hopefulness. If they are fairly open about what has and hasn't worked for them, they may provide a good role model for you and your partner.

Actively Seek
Solutions to Problems

Begin quite consciously and deliberately to work on your problem or problems once identified. One of you may feel more strongly about the problem than the other, but it is still worth putting effort into developing some kind of strategy or plan to work away at the problem. Examples of conscious, deliberate, and intentional perseverance might be the following: Trying to get home a bit earlier from your working day to be with your spouse and children; not drinking during the week but only on weekends; dividing up the domestic chores so that each of you feel that the workload is more evenly distributed; taking turns booking the baby-sitter and planning an activity for your night out together; volunteering that you are feeling upset about something and need to discuss it rather than withdrawing into a cold, angry silence; planning a vacation together; taking turns reading your child a story at bedtime; and sitting down together and planning a budget.

The underlying motive and intention of any of the above examples of working at problems are that you and your spouse are in agreement that something is amiss and that there is something to be gained by trying to change one's own behavior. A better level of communication, harmony, and closeness are the possible benefits.

What do you do if you and your spouse simply can't agree about the nature of the problem or problems? I suggest that you try to accept this difference in good faith. Unfortunately, too many couples debate and argue about their identified problems without reaching any kind of consensus. They then get into secondary conflicts over power and control, and meanwhile, neither makes any effort to change the original annoying behavior.

Programs and Workshops

Give some thought to attending a marital enrichment program in your community. The vast majority of individuals who have returned from a marital enrichment workshop, whether it's an evening or a weekend, feel that it was a very worthwhile, if not phenomenal, experience. These meetings are generally meant to be for enhancement of the marriage and for renewal, not for couples who are in serious marital trouble. They are predicated on the premise that *all* marriages need renewal, growth, and new learning from time to time. It is also assumed that both parties will be interested in attending and will try to keep an open mind to what is offered.

Marital enrichment courses are offered by most of the major religions and will vary a great deal in terms of the prominence of religious dogma in the format. Secular marital enrichment experiences are offered by community colleges, universities, and private groups. They are usually conducted by social workers, psychologists, or marital/family therapists who have a special interest and expertise in enhancing couples' communication, functioning, and solidarity. There are usually group sessions wherein general principles are discussed and then individual couples work on assignments and exercises on their own. Couples are not expected to disclose their personal and interpersonal issues with the other couples attending.

Some marital enrichment workshops will spend part of the time, or the entire time, on a particular theme. Some of these themes may be of particular interest to you and your spouse. Examples might include

- What do women want?
- What do men want?
- What works and doesn't work in stepfamilies?
- How to cope with your extended family
- Enhancing intimacy in your marriage
- Two-paycheck marriages
- Working on your marriage as retirement approaches

Do Some Reading About Marriage

Women tend to be much more interested in reading about marriage than men, although there are some glaring exceptions. In fact, maybe you've had the experience of coming across an interesting article in a magazine or reading a book that you think is helpful. You take the time to highlight some passages in the article or put it aside for your husband to read, but days and weeks pass without his commenting on it. You find that he hasn't read it and he gives you some sort of excuse that he hasn't had time. Actually, the truth is that he isn't interested.

Men's general reluctance or disinterest in reading about marriage is probably rooted in the historical fact that tending to the health of a marriage was the woman's job. The whole notion of "working at" your marriage and learning to communicate better is all quite recent, that is, only in the past few decades. Even that is not universally accepted. For many couples, getting married is a religious and legal exercise with only lip service paid to its quality and ways of enhancing that quality. Many married people, and especially men, ascribe to the oversimplified notion that being a good provider, being faithful, and watching one's health are all that are necessary for marital happiness. So reading books about marriage is unnecessary, if not simply silly. I recommend that both of you go to the library or bookstore and browse through books *together*.

How Do We Know if We Need Professional Help?

I suggest that you and your spouse try some of the above suggestions, the ones that apply to you and that seem reasonable. Give yourselves a few weeks or even a few months to work on changing things. You should certainly be able to tell during a reasonable time interval if things are beginning to improve, if things are beginning to shift. Perhaps you'll feel calmer. Perhaps you'll feel happier. Perhaps you'll notice that you and your partner seem to be communicating more easily. You may also find that your communication is more effective and that you are solving problems much easier, and faster. And you might find that you like each other again.

Because there is a cyclical pattern to marital distress, you may not quite trust the improvement that you and your spouse are making. Although that is certainly understandable, my suggestion is that you wait it out and keep applying the principles and suggestions mentioned above. If you go several months without a bad period, or only minor upsets, then I would say you are doing very well.

Don't despair if things don't seem to be improving, or seem to be worsening, despite your best intentions and best efforts. Also don't despair if things seem very slow or equivocal. And try not to associate seeking professional help with failure. You may be misjudging the complicated nature of your problem and what appears on the surface to be quite simple and quite straightforward may not be so. There are other variables related to other stressors in your life or your background or your spouse's background, and you will not always be able to untangle and resolve every problem. What you may find is that you and your spouse are going around in circles or you are becoming entangled or embroiled in issues from which you cannot see your way clear. Usually what this means is that the problem is the tip of the iceberg, with origins going back to your early months or years together, or perhaps even further, into your respective childhoods and the homes in which you were raised. These issues probably won't be visible to you, only to the eye of a trained observer and experienced therapist.

You and your partner may have a short list of problems or subjects that you just can't discuss, despite all the suggestions made above. In fact, the two of you may have been applying those actions on your own for years without success. You will need to accept, for the time

---

She Says . . .

"My husband and I are like very good friends. There's no spark, no sexual chemistry anymore. I think we should still feel sensual, even though we've been together a long time."

This is a very common complaint from couples who have been together for a while. At one end of the spectrum are couples who are just a bit bogged down with each other—their marriages are devitalized. At the other end are couples who are quite estranged emotionally and certainly erotically, so indeed they are like good friends. Whether they remain together is highly individual.

In a devitalized marriage, the two individuals have been so busy that intimate time as a couple has been sacrificed or "relegated to the back burner." When they do take the time to make love, they may find it rather strained or even impossible because the experience feels a bit foreign and frightening. Hence, they conclude, "Well, we're good friends, and we have common goals. We're just not really lovers anymore."

being, that those are problems that are difficult and complicated and are impossible for the two of you to discuss and work out with each other on your own. Further, because each of you has been so frustrated about these problems, you may feel a range of other emotions such as hurt, anger, a sense of being attacked, betrayal, and shame. These emotions may have prevented any further attempts to get these problems resolved. There are many examples of problems that couples find difficult to discuss: sexual concerns (very common, no matter how open or sophisticated either of you might be about your sexuality), the guidance and disciplining of children if you and your spouse are in a stepfamily, defensiveness about excessive drinking in your partner, unresolved feelings about an unexpected pregnancy or a therapeutic abortion, clogged communication regarding a previous extramarital affair, bisexuality in either you or your spouse, your relationship with an ex-partner, and the changing sex roles of women and men in the workplace and in the home. Many of these topics are more easily raised, discussed, debated, and resolved in the therapist's office and in a neutral setting with guidance and assistance.

If things at home have gotten very bad, or if things are escalating quickly, causing a lot of tension, arguing, yelling, screaming, or threats about separating or any physical violence, try to arrange for a visit with a marital therapist as quickly as possible. Many couples find that even if they have to wait a few days or a few weeks to see someone, they will feel significantly better and the tension will diminish simply because they have come to a decision to seek professional help. Even if the two of you have made a decision to separate, I still strongly suggest that you book a consultation visit with a marital therapist. His or her experienced counsel will assist you in reinforcing your decision (if he or she agrees with your decision), or there may be a suggestion that the two of you try to delay your separation. Your therapist may feel that a decision to separate is premature and perhaps unnecessary.

Very often a trial of marital therapy can be illuminating. It is possible that each of you may be overreacting to your unhappiness and disaffection with each other. Therefore, separation will provide relief, but your decision still may be ill-conceived or premature. With a trial of marital therapy, the therapist might suggest that you slow down your plans to separate. While you are doing this, the anger and frustration you feel toward each other may be released, and it is quite possible that submerged and camouflaged positive feelings may return. If this occurs, you may find that you want to reconsider separating.

Even if your marriage is over and separation is both necessary and inevitable, slowing it down gives you and your spouse much more time to prepare yourselves, both physically and psychologically. You may need time to discuss which one is going to move out and where, who is staying with the children, what to do about your furnishings, and your arrangement regarding joint monies until something can be done legally. Delaying a separation gives you more time to consider these things and to grieve and prepare yourself for being on your own. Even if you feel that you don't need the time because you have been working on this for months or years on your own, your partner may need the time to work through strong feelings such as abandonment, rage, hurt, and shame and feelings of failure, guilt, and terror at being on one's own.

There are many other reasons for seeing a marital therapist even if you and your spouse have made a decision to separate. Your decision to live apart will be validated, the fact that your marriage is beyond repair will be affirmed (so that you can stop blaming yourself or each other for not trying hard enough), and the act of separating will be accepted as a reality. Marital therapists don't simply help people fix up their marriages; they also help people separate with less pain and more dignity.

TEN

Basic Information About Marital Therapy

The evidence that marital therapy is effective is not simply based on the vast number of people who can attest to that; there is now a significant body of scientific literature supporting its effectiveness for couples in distress. It's very helpful to sit down with someone who is not living your marriage, someone who can objectively interpret what's happening.

Here is a caution, however. Some couples find that their situation gets worse before it gets better, and what this usually indicates is the presence of unresolved buried issues. These must be uncovered and dealt with before you and your spouse can move on to settle your current difficulties. Your therapist should be watching for this and will be able to help you understand what is taking place.

Also keep in mind that the focus in therapy tends to be on what is *not* working as opposed to what *is* working. Therefore, try not to lose sight of the fact that in many ways, perhaps in most ways, you and your spouse may get along very well. There are simply pockets and areas of discord and resentment that need resolution. Your attempts to live with them and to "agree to disagree" have not worked—and your attempts to sweep them under the carpet have been futile.

If your marital issues are irreconcilable, if there is very little binding the two of you together, and if separation can't be prevented, you may feel worse rather than better with therapy. But this will not go on forever, and when or if the two of you come to an agreement about separation, the decision in itself will give you some relief. You will feel better again for reasons different from those among couples who will be staying together, but you will be feeling better, nonetheless.

Whom to See

A range of professional people provide marital therapy services. It can be quite confusing for people to know whether they should be seeing their family doctor, someone in the clergy, a psychologist, a social worker, a "marriage counselor," or a psychiatrist. I'll come to the specifics of each of these disciplines in a moment.

Another consideration that you should keep in mind is whether your concerns are general and are ones that a range of marital therapists are experienced treating on an everyday basis. If you have a specific complaint that may be unusual, or one that requires a specific type of marital therapy approach, then it is best to seek out someone in your community who does that particular kind of work. Here are some examples of what I mean:

- One or both of you may have some kind of specific sexual dysfunction
- Your spouse is bisexual, or possibly gay
- One or both of you are alcoholic
- You are part of a stepfamily
- You are a battered spouse
- You are HIV positive or have AIDS
- Your husband is a cross-dresser (dresses up in women's clothes), and this is very hard for you to accept and live with in your marriage

- Your marriage was fine until your daughter told you that she is lesbian, and now all the two of you do is fight and blame each other
- You have breast cancer and your husband has withdrawn from you and refuses to discuss it
- Your husband has bipolar illness, and you would like to see someone who has an understanding about this illness

If you live in a small community, you may have very few options and may be obliged to see someone who does general marital therapy. However, this may be more beneficial than you believe because that individual may be able to use very general skills with you that will help a great deal. He or she may then be able to refer you on to a specialist in another community who has expertise in dealing with the kinds of problems the two of you are experiencing. Having said that, if you happen to work in the mental health field yourself, or your spouse does, you may be reluctant to see a marital therapist in your community because your paths may cross professionally. In this case you may wish to seek marital therapy in a nearby community.

When you come to the stage of recognizing and accepting that the two of you need to see a marital therapist, try to identify some of the difficult issues. What's important is that you consider both your own needs and preferences as well as your spouse's needs and preferences. What would each of you expect or want from the therapist? Are your goals and expectations quite similar, or are they very different? Would your spouse accept or reject the therapist or a particular kind of therapist that you would like to see? Are you able to determine the kind of person with whom your spouse might be the most comfortable and most trusting? Is there anything that you can do to make this decision about seeing someone, and the process of executing it, less threatening for your spouse and, ultimately, for yourself? What I've just described is not that easy in actual practice, but that said, it is important to try to talk with each other as much as you can about going to see a professional.

Many couples come to see me because one partner has done all of the work in setting it up. It's not unusual for the spouse to feel dragged along, bullied into coming, or threatened in some way.

However, this may be the way you operate in your marriage on a regular basis anyway, so that how you get to marital therapy is a metaphor of how you get through life together, with one person making the decisions and leading the way and the other tagging along.

Let me say a few words about the various kinds of professionals who do marital therapy.

Family Physicians

Often couples will turn to their family doctor first if they are having marital troubles, or to their primary care physician, internist, or other medical specialist. Your family doctor is in a unique position to assist you in finding help for your marital trouble because this may be one professional with whom you have cultivated a trusting relationship. He or she may have been your family physician for some time, has looked after you, perhaps has delivered your children, and may also be your partner's and your children's doctor.

Your family physician may be the first one to wonder if you are having marital distress. Perhaps you've come to the office with a range of physical symptoms for which no organic basis can be found, and your family doctor begins to wonder what might be causing your distress. At that point you may be asked about your marriage, and your doctor should be able to refer you and your spouse to someone who does marital therapy. Knowing that your doctor is sending you to a professional who is trusted and respected should ease some of your anxiety about going for help.

I suggest that if you have a family physician, you speak to that person if you are having concerns about your marriage. Your doctor should be there to listen, to ask you questions, to get some idea of the severity of your concerns, to diagnose and treat any complicating or additional problems, to provide comfort and reassurance, and to discuss marital therapy options with you. If your partner is not a patient of your family physician, you might consider bringing him or her along with you—if not to the first visit, certainly to the second. A meeting like this enables your family physician to sit with both of you and explain treatment.

Religious Counselors

If you are religiously oriented or affiliated, you may wish to consult your minister, priest, rabbi, imam, or other spiritual guide about your marriage. Your clergyperson may be able to give you specific counseling for your difficulties or a recommendation to see another professional, depending on your needs and whether he or she is trained in marital therapy.

Whether you are comfortable speaking to the clergy will depend on your relationship with that person, how much you trust him or her, how private you are about such matters, and the degree to which you want to keep your marital concerns separate from your involvement in your religion. My impression, however, is that many people reject the notion of meeting with their clergyperson without a good basis for that rejection. At a time of significant marital crisis, your spiritual leader or adviser can be very comforting and give you a sense of perspective on your situation.

These days it is highly unusual for a member of the clergy to admonish people for having marital difficulty. In fact, most of them understand that many marriages do not and cannot work, and they can be very supportive of the need to separate if at least one attempt at marital therapy has been made. Although people fear this, it is highly uncommon nowadays for people to come away from a meeting with their spiritual leader feeling more guilty than when they went in.

In addition, most major religions have some type of ongoing support group or social network for members who are separated or divorced. This option not only is therapeutically useful but is also one way of combating the stigma that some people feel about being divorced.

Professional Therapists

Nonmedical therapists make up the bulk of professionals who do marital therapy. Some are marriage counselors, and some have degrees in psychology, social work, or nursing. The training of nonmedical therapists varies tremendously, from no postsecondary education to the requirement of a doctorate. The best therapists will have at least a master's degree or a doctorate, will be licensed to perform marital therapy, and will be registered with the local branch of their national professional association. Beyond that, some will have done further training in marital and family therapy, and will belong to one or more national or international organizations (see Appendix). It is essential that you ask your therapist what his or her credentials are regarding training and membership in professional associations and societies.

You may prefer to see a nonmedical therapist for several reasons. You might feel that a physician therapist, either a family physician, internist, or psychiatrist, might tend to underestimate the severity of your difficulty and feel that your concerns are not worthy of time and attention. You might also feel that medical therapists are not as well trained in psychological, marital, and family matters because so much of their education has been in the biological sciences as opposed to the psychological and social sciences. You might also be fearful that a therapist who is a physician, especially a psychiatrist, will label you with a psychiatric diagnosis and treat you with medication like tranquilizers and antidepressants instead of with talk therapy. In fact, if you did suffer from a major psychiatric illness at one time earlier in your life that required medication or hospitalization, you may be especially concerned about psychiatric labeling and medication.

I have been quite deliberate in referring to the situations above as fear related. Depending on the specifics of your situation, your fear may be entirely appropriate and very real, but you could also be experiencing symptoms of a psychiatric illness or addiction. This will affect your thinking, your mood, and your judgment, thereby giving you a perception of, or actually causing, marital unhappiness and conflict. In this case, you could indeed benefit from seeing or being referred to a medical therapist.

Psychiatrists

Because psychiatrists are physicians who have completed medical training, they can offer you a comprehensive assessment of your marriage and suggest a range of treatment options. Seeing a psychiatrist may be particularly helpful if you are having numerous symptoms, such as feeling anxious, not sleeping well, depressed mood, or changed appetite. A psychiatrist can determine if you have a clinical illness and need to receive individual treatment along with, or instead of, marital therapy. A psychiatrist will discuss medication with you if he or she feels that is necessary.

A psychiatrist should also be able to help you sort out whether your marriage is making you ill, your illness is affecting your marriage, or if there is a bit of both going on. If your psychiatrist feels that you're having symptoms because you are distressed about your marriage, then the best approach is for you and your spouse to see someone together. If, on the other hand, you and your spouse are having difficulty because you are suffering from quite a severe depression, then the psychiatrist may want to treat this first and see if your marriage improves once your mood improves.

If you are living with some type of medical problem such as high blood pressure, diabetes, migraine headaches, or arthritis, a psychiatrist will have an understanding of how these illnesses affect people

She Says . . .

"He's got a temper. He's never hit me, but I tell him he scares me sometimes."

This is an important subject to get resolved because if his temper doesn't get talked about, and acknowledged, his wife will feel controlled by it. That is, not only will she remain frightened by her husband when he's upset, she will do everything in her power *not* to provoke him. This is hard to do, if not impossible, but more importantly, it is no way to live in a relationship and is morally repugnant.

Is this man embarrassed, worried, or disgusted by his outbursts, and is he motivated to do something about them? Because with some individual therapy and one or more visits with his wife, he probably can. It is more ominous if this man does not see this as his problem but sees it as his wife's. Verbal or emotional violence, and its impact on others, is as serious and as damaging as physical battering. But many men and women do not like to hear that words hit as hard as a fist.

psychologically and how they can affect marriage. If you are on medication, a psychiatrist will be able to determine if your medication is affecting your mood, sexual functioning, anxiety level, or your ability to sleep. All of these can affect marital communication.

Even though a psychiatrist may be in an advantageous position to provide a comprehensive assessment of your situation, he or she may not have training in marital therapy and may suggest individuals in the community whom you and your spouse could see.

There are situations in which family therapy might be indicated. Usually this is recommended to couples by a child or adolescent psychiatrist who has been asked to assess or treat one of the children. That person may feel that the best approach is to see the entire family and will recommend that course of action to you. Some family therapists also do marital therapy; it may be helpful to see a therapist with that specific training because he or she may want the children to come in at some point, or from time to time. You may find that to be very helpful.

Different Approaches to Marital Therapy

You may be curious about the theoretical training and orientation of your therapist because you may have some ideas yourself as to the kind of approach you feel the two of you need or from which you can benefit. Or perhaps you had treatment before as a couple by someone of a particular theoretical orientation and you feel that you went as far as you could go with that person. Indeed, it might have been helpful but there are still some difficulties that the two of you feel need resolution and perhaps a different approach.

At the risk of oversimplification, there are three theoretical schools that have contributed to our understanding of marriage and marital therapy: *behavioral, systems,* and *psychoanalytic-psychodynamic.* Let me briefly describe each of them.

Behavioral Approach

The behavioral approach to marital therapy is based in the theory of learning. Your therapist will help the two of you identify the ways in which you and your spouse interact that are not working, that are unsuccessful and causing conflict. Your therapist will then teach the two of you some new ways of interacting with each other. A simple example: It annoys you that your husband doesn't wash around the sink in the mornings after shaving. He, on the other hand, gets very annoyed when you keep him waiting when the two of you are going out to the theater. Your therapist will try to help each of you work on changing your own behavior over an agreed-upon period, say 2 to 4 weeks. Coupled with this, your therapist will also help each of you toward negotiating some type of specific and concrete reward for changing your behavior. You agree to make a special candlelit dinner once every 2 weeks; he agrees to let you sleep in on Sunday mornings while he takes the kids to the park.

Systems Approach

This approach to marital conflict is based on the premise that if one family member makes a change, this is followed by a change somewhere else in the family system. For example, your husband is alcoholic and he consents to go for treatment and begins to improve. But unless you get some help yourself, you may not be as happy with his changed behavior and attitude as you had originally thought you would be. Or you may find yourself reacting in a way that makes you question if you might have been making his problem with alcohol worse. This is called *codependency* or *enabling* and is noted in families in which one or more members are alcoholic.

Psychoanalytic-Psychodynamic Approach

The psychoanalytic-psychodynamic perspective is based on the premise that we are truly the products of our past and that when we marry, when we interact with our spouse, and whom we marry are highly determined by the home in which we grew up and the relationship we had with our parents and siblings. There may be a lesser or greater amount of inner conflict experienced by one or both partners, which may then be brought into the marriage.

Here are two examples: If you find yourself becoming shaky or having palpitations when your husband raises his voice, this may be because your father often yelled at your mother while you were growing up and you hated it. Or it may be that your father yelled at you, and at these moments in your marriage, your husband reminds you of your father. Another example is if you find yourself getting panicky when you and your spouse argue. This might be because you have a fear of abandonment. You are afraid that your spouse might leave you, even though you've been assured that leaving is the furthest thing from his or her mind. This also comes from your background. Perhaps your parents fought a lot and you feared they would separate. Maybe they did separate, and you found that extremely difficult.

Other Approaches

In addition to these three basic theoretical orientations, there are many other schools of thought that may contribute to your therapist's approach. Many therapists are multidimensional in their approach to couples and integrate the various types of therapy. You and your spouse may respond best to a certain approach at one time and a different approach at another. It may be that certain of your problems are best managed with a particular approach, whereas other problems are best treated with another.

Another way of classifying marital therapy is according to the format used by the therapist. The most common format is *conjoint therapy*, meaning that your therapist meets with the two of you together at the same time. Some therapists are very orthodox about this approach and refuse to see either partner in the marriage on their own. Their approach is to always see the two of you together to assist you as best they can with making self-disclosures and with improving communication. Therapists like this are not interested in hearing secrets from either one of you. They are only interested in the communications that you are willing to talk about with each other in their presence.

Most therapists who use a conjoint approach are not this rigid. A conjoint approach may be their preferred mode of treatment, but they will want to see each of you alone at the beginning of treatment, usually after the first conjoint visit, for at least one visit. The purpose of these individual visits is to enable the therapist to learn details about your personal and family history. Then some time later, after a series of conjoint visits, your therapist may wish to meet with each of you alone again. Should either of you request to meet with the therapist alone, he or she will honor that, provided that both you and your spouse are comfortable with the request.

Another type of marital therapy is what is called *concurrent marital therapy*. In this approach, your therapist is looking after both of you in individual treatment. From time to time your therapist may see the two of you together, but most of the visits will be individual ones as each of you explores your individual lives and comes to better understand yourself.

Some therapists practice what is called *collaborative therapy*. In this approach, you are each in individual therapy but with different therapists. The therapists, with your permission, keep in touch with each other and collaborate over what is going on in your individual respective therapies.

Another form of marital therapy is *cotherapy*. Cotherapy occurs when two therapists, who are usually of the opposite sex, work together and treat the two of you conjointly. The advantages of this kind of therapy are twofold: Each of you will feel that you have a representative in the therapy from your own gender, and secondly, your cotherapists may even model a form of mutually respectful communication that could be of interest to, or a learning experience for, the two of you.

And finally, some therapists, either on their own or with a cotherapist, run *couples groups*. These groups are usually made up of anywhere from three to five couples who meet on a regular basis for group therapy. The issues discussed may be common to many couples, or it is possible that the group is composed of couples who are all struggling with the same kinds of issues.

The Integrated Model of Treatment

I want to say a few words about the value of an integrated model of therapy. There are many ways to define integrated therapy, but I am restricting my definition here to the use of both a conjoint and individual treatment approach. I find that with some couples it can be very beneficial to begin therapy with a course of conjoint work for several weeks, followed by a course of individual treatment for one or both of the individuals, followed by conjoint work again in an alternating and reciprocal pattern as necessary. There is a dynamic interplay between these two approaches. The conjoint visits help identify the major areas of conflict for the couple, and this can also be the best forum for resolving many of these conflicts.

However, there may be more deeply buried conflicts in one or both of the individuals that are best uncovered and worked through in individual therapy. It's interesting to hear from my patients' statements such as the following:

> I have found it very helpful to have this series of individual sessions with you. I couldn't have done this work at the beginning because I really didn't know what my problems were at that time. Also, I think I would have found working on these issues by myself rather threatening.

In other words, this more intensive one-on-one psychotherapy was really not possible without the earlier conjoint work, and the later conjoint work really can't proceed without the intervening individual work.

Even if you or your partner is hesitant to look for or to begin individual therapy, I suggest that you do some conjoint work with a couples therapist. This will help to settle things down in terms of the conflicts you are experiencing and may soothe the atmosphere at home. More important, each of you will get an opportunity to establish some rapport with the therapist. As the interaction between your therapist and each of you evolves, you'll get a chance to observe, to assess, and to decide how much you trust and respect your therapist's competence. All the while, you will be making a determination as to how comfortable, willing, or interested you are in individual treatment.

I find that men especially can benefit from this sequencing of individual therapy following a course of conjoint therapy. Because men are so often the reluctant partners in going for therapy, this approach gives them an opportunity to "buy time" while they make a decision to look inward and explore some of their own issues that are contributing to their life difficulties.

How Long Is the Treatment?

How long does marital therapy take? Most experiences are relatively brief, that is, anywhere from 6 to 12 visits, usually 1 hour in length and scheduled once a week or once every 2 weeks. That said, your situation may not necessarily lend itself to this kind of conventional or predictable "package." But don't worry if your course of therapy goes on longer. Some couples simply need a longer period to get to know their therapist and to have a sense that they are forging a therapeutic relationship. Some also have deep-seated underlying issues, including sexual concerns, which are harder to talk about and may not surface for several weeks. Certain couples prefer a longer period between visits, say 3 to 4 weeks, because a lot comes out in one visit and it takes a while to process the feelings and communications that take place in the therapist's office.

Furthermore, the visits may be emotionally upsetting or draining, and you may want more time before you go back to the therapist. Some people simply want more time between visits to work on things so that they get a feeling of change. And finally, some couples need to experiment with different approaches and formats at different times with their therapist before certain personal and interpersonal problems surface and are ready to be tackled.

ELEVEN
Marital Therapy
Benefits and Barriers

The Benefits of Professional Help

Simply Talking to Someone Objective

When you think of it, doesn't it make sense to talk to a professional person about something as important as your marriage, your mental health, or the mental health of your family members? The therapist you see will likely be trained in a specific discipline or will be experienced in treating distressed couples—and he or she will be objective and neutral without being cold and mechanical. The objectivity a therapist offers is something that your friends and family can't provide because they have an emotional attachment to you.

Your therapist should be someone who observes well, listens carefully, and can sort through the many layers of conflict from your background, your spouse's background, and your early weeks or years together. The therapist should also be a good diagnostician—not just someone who can diagnose your marital conflict, but someone who can diagnose associated illness in each of you and whether this illness is a cause of your marital difficulty, a result of it, or both.

Marital therapists use their training and skills to perceive and clarify issues that may be confusing to you. They sort out communication

problems that characterize your relationship and prompt and rein-
force feelings or, alternately, help to put a "lid" on feelings when it
seems necessary. They watch for and decide with you if you or your
spouse could benefit from more intensive treatment like individual
therapy, medication, or even hospitalization if mental functioning is quite compromised.

As I mentioned earlier, a well-trained and experienced professional should be able to offer you assistance, guidance, and hope. And I mean hope here in a very general sense, that the two of you will get through this very difficult time in your lives and will be better people for it, whether you remain together or not. All good therapy is based on the premise of trust, and you should be able to believe that your therapist is trustworthy and has the best interests of each of you at heart. A good therapist does not take sides. In fact, if you feel that your therapist is taking your side against your spouse, or your spouse's side against you, it is critical that you bring it up directly. You may not recognize it in a particular visit, but if that feeling persists (even if it is not shared by your spouse), I strongly suggest that you bring it up with your therapist

She Says, He Says . . .

She says: "I'm very lonely. I just don't know if he loves me anymore."

He says: "I'm noticing other women a lot these days. I'm not sure what this means, but it scares me."

This woman's concern is very telling; it epitomizes her frustration, boredom, and sense of emptiness with her husband. Unfortunately, this situation is all too common and it is serious. What troubles me is that often these women are made to feel that they are just whining and dependent, that they need to make more of a life of their own and look less to their husbands for attention. I see far too many women who have been made to feel that they alone are the problem when, in fact, they are only one of two players in a marital dynamic of blocked communication and isolation.

Most people in marriage find themselves attracted to others throughout the life cycle.

However, when feelings for someone else become very strong or persistent, this usually says something about the marriage, more specifically, about what this man is not receiving from his spouse.

He should ask himself, "Am I sitting on anger toward my wife and not letting her know?" If he is, his marriage may actually be fine. But if he doesn't feel any anger but just feels somewhat neutral or detached, his feelings of attraction toward other(s) may represent loneliness and estrangement that possibly have been building for some time, probably years.

at the next visit. If you don't, treatment cannot and will not work, and you will be wasting your time and money.

There is something distinctly and uniquely advantageous about forming a working relationship with your therapist. It is very different from a personal friendship, although it is characterized by similar aspects such as mutual respect, warmth, fondness, responsibility, and of course trust. One important difference is that you and your spouse will be "baring your souls" but your therapist will not.

Statements like the following from my practice are very common:

- "It's a relief to come here to talk with you about these problems. Some of them are problems that we have discussed with our close friends, but both of us think they must be sick of hearing about our difficulties. Coming here, we don't have to worry about wearing out or alienating our friends."
- "Our friends are wonderful and they are very supportive, but they unfortunately tend to take my side against my spouse."
- "You seem to have a very different take on us. In fact, you're the only person we've talked to who seems to understand why we're still together, why we're not divorced."
- "You haven't really said anything that is new to us or anything that we didn't already know, but because you're a professional, we find that we listen to you, certainly a lot more than we listen to each other."
- "It's a great relief to me that we don't know you personally or that our paths don't cross socially. I feel that I can be really honest here and open up to you without fearing that you are judging us. It's less embarrassing than talking to my family and my friends."

Things Change Faster

Living with marital conflict or unhappiness can prove demoralizing and tiring. Therapy speeds up the process of beginning to feel better again. You also begin to think more clearly, to become more clear in your decision making, and, most important, to become ready to take action. This change in approach and attitude is critical (and also usually welcome!) when you've been beleaguered with marital worries for some time, or if you live with ambivalence about what to do, or if you are essentially paralyzed into inactivity by feeling so guilty and despondent. Many couples can actually identify the inner feeling of being stuck or in a stalemate.

Sharing the Responsibility

One of the features of the doctor-patient relationship, or therapist-patient relationship, is transferring at least part of the responsibility you are bearing onto someone else. This is part of the therapeutic contract and is to be expected. I am talking not about complete responsibility being shifted from yourselves onto the therapist but only about a partial transfer of some of the weight with which you are living. Again, this doesn't mean that the therapist actually takes on your burdens, but it does mean that he or she is there to assist you, guide you, and attempt to uncover solutions with you. I believe that all individuals and couples understand that the responsibility for their marriage rests with each of them and that ultimately they have to make their decisions themselves.

When you transfer some of the responsibility for your marital difficulty to your therapist, there are certain factors in operation. First of all, you and your spouse have probably been feeling overwhelmed or confused, and second, you should be able to perceive and expect a sense of hope and strength in your therapist. This will allow you to trust and let go a little.

Dealing With Your Guilt

Most people who are experiencing marital difficulty feel guilty that, despite their best efforts, things don't feel very good. There is a tendency for self-blame, especially if you're not able to do things in a way you think would be better. This is compounded if you have children, especially young children. Most parents feel it is unfair for their kids to live in a home in which their mom and dad are not happy. If there's tension, arguing, or fighting within earshot of the children or in their presence, this compounds the guilt. If the tension and unhappiness are severe and there are threats of separation or there is an actual decision to separate, this leads to another layer of guilt. This is the guilt associated with the parents' notion of failure in letting themselves, their children, and their families down.

In situations in which only one partner wants the separation, that person usually feels very guilty. It is exacerbated if there are no major or glaring shortcomings in the partner that are visible on the surface. Very often, in the early stages, the reasons for separating make sense only to the partner who wants out or to his or her close friends. It can take much longer for family and others to see the relief that accrues with being separated. And it is especially difficult to leave someone who desperately loves you and has absolutely no desire to have the marriage end.

If you're struggling with guilt, or if you're finding it overwhelming, it can be extremely helpful to talk with a therapist. You'll feel relief in talking about your problems and "getting things off your chest." It also helps to allay your guilt when your therapist can validate what you are experiencing as completely understandable, and also as completely normal, given your situation and the specifics of your marital unrest.

Your therapist will try to assist the two of you in whatever way possible with your specific problems by helping to decrease the tension and arguing at home, perhaps suggesting ways the two of you can talk with your children about what is going on and helping you explain to them that you are both trying to do something about this and that you are seeing a marital therapist.

Fighting Demoralization

Demoralization is common when things aren't going well in a marriage. It is a perfectly understandable consequence of days, weeks, months, and years of friction, misunderstanding, and unhappiness. It's embodied by such statements as "I don't care anymore," "I'm fed up," "I'm worn out," "I've lost my morale," "This isn't worth it."

Talking to a marital therapist who is used to dealing with couples' problems can give you a bit of a different perspective. It's possible that your situation isn't nearly as bad as you view it. Not to make light of what you're feeling, but you may not be aware of why things are as stuck as they seem to be, nor might you be aware of different kinds of communication strategies and other options. Therefore, it may be startling to hear your therapist sum up, at the end of your first visit, with statements like these:

- "Well, I agree that things look very bad; however, let us work together for a while and see what happens. I think we'll have a better idea of where your marriage is heading a month from now."
- "I know that the two of you feel terrible about what's going on at home, but my sense is that you both love each other a lot and are very committed to making your marriage work. Let's have a few visits together and see if you are able to regain at least some of that good feeling that you used to have for each other."
- "I can see that you're both very unhappy and that you can't go on living like this the way things are. However, given the amount of stress in your lives, it's amazing that you're coping as well as you are. The unhappiness that you're feeling, and your tense communication with each other, is very common in couples who have had a death in the family, a change of job, and a brush with cancer all in 1 year. Don't make any impulsive decisions about your marriage until I've had an opportunity to work with both of you over the next couple of months, and we'll review where things are then."

The Reluctant Spouse

Spousal resistance to marital therapy is very common. Many individuals go to their family doctor, their clergyperson, or their therapist with vague complaints of unrest or unhappiness. These can indicate a marital problem, and therapy may be suggested by the professional. But when they bring this information home, their spouse refuses to go with them to see someone. In many homes, the marital problem is obvious to both partners, yet one of them absolutely refuses to go for help. Many of these people will eventually go for help with their partners but not until the marriage is on its last legs, separation is imminent, or separation has already taken place.

Why is this? Why do people feel so resistant to marital therapy? In an attempt to shed light on this phenomenon, I will outline several of the most common factors in the following sections. I will explain, at least partially, the attitude and behavior of the so-called reluctant spouse, who is often labeled as selfish, uncaring, rigid, falsely proud, unmotivated, or simply lazy. Some spouses fit these descriptions, but in my experience they are in the minority.

Privacy

Some people are just very, very private; they don't open up easily with anyone, including their spouse. Therefore, they are not going to talk easily to a complete stranger, even if that person is a professional. They may be even less likely to talk in a self-disclosing way in the presence of their spouse.

One's sense of privacy may actually be a lifelong trait that goes back to childhood and possibly into the family as well. There can be both genetic and environmental factors involved. In some cases, these same people are prone to mistrustfulness, suspicion, or frank paranoid thinking.

Others are private because they are simply shy, they do not have healthy self-esteem, or they live with feelings of unworthiness. Some people don't open up easily because their privacy has been betrayed in the past on a number of occasions; hence, they have developed a sense that people can't be trusted, especially with very personal information. And finally, some people are quite private because when they have been open and forthcoming, they have been ridiculed or put down so much that they have adopted a posture of playing it safe and saying nothing, or very little.

Self-Reliance

Many people define themselves as self-reliant—they are used to solving their own problems and have always functioned that way. In fact, most of the time this has worked well for them and they, in turn, take pride in their independence and in their self-sufficiency. Throughout my career as a psychiatrist, I've been amazed at the number of people I have met as patients who are extremely resourceful. They outline terrible histories of unhappy childhoods, all kinds of personal and family losses, and many other stressful times in their lives when they've received virtually no help. Furthermore, these same individuals have often coped through periods in their lives completely on their own and with a great deal of courage and determination. They have developed and used a range of coping strategies that have served them well: a rugged determination to carry on, a fighting spirit, an abhorrence for self-pity, a phenomenal ability to concentrate on positive thoughts (and to push away the negative), a capacity for reflection, and a philosophy of hope.

These are wonderful skills, and they are rooted in individualism. However, these same skills and strategies do not work nearly as well with marital difficulty. They may be useful in allowing people to recognize and understand what the issues are, but they will not be helpful in trying to overcome them. Dialogue and discussion are so fundamental in solving marital differences and unhappiness that the open approach may not be easy for the rugged individualist. For these people, it is exactly this shared communication that is lacking in their marriage. And it is longed for by their partners. In fact, these same individuals may put down marital therapy as a complete waste of their, and the therapist's, time.

These individuals tend to do something else that is anathema to one-on-one communication. They trivialize their marital discord by comparing it with the major events in their life that have been painful and traumatic, and that they have overcome. Or they compare marital difficulties with the major crises that are occurring at any one time on a global basis, for example, war, famine, poverty, or AIDS. By advancing these kinds of comparisons, they not only are resisting engagement in marital therapy but are also shutting out the worries and fears of their spouses.

Ineffective Previous Treatment

If you or your spouse has had an earlier experience with a therapist that was not helpful, or worse, destructive, you will not want to rush back into therapy again. Even if this happened many years ago, the memory of it may still be quite strong. If you agree or your spouse agrees to try some form of help again, one or both of you may have a lot of trouble getting through your feelings of wariness, mistrust, or simple lack of enthusiasm.

Sometimes the fallout from a negative therapy experience can be quite pervasive. You may feel negative toward all mental health professionals or only specific disciplines. Or you may be negative about mental health professionals of a particular sex: you have had it with women therapists but are willing to try a male therapist (or vice versa). And sometimes it doesn't matter whether the previous negative treatment experience was individual therapy, as part of a couple, or in your current or previous relationship.

It is very upsetting to harbor negative feelings from a previous therapy experience. It is also easy to see how these perceptions and feelings can leave people feeling wary and nervous about engaging in treatment again. If you are married to someone who is resistant to marital therapy, it would be wise to talk about any earlier therapy experiences.

Psychiatric Illness

If you and your partner are going to see a psychiatrist for marital therapy, you may be anxious about the process because of your background. For instance, if either of your parents, any siblings, or other relatives who are close to you have suffered from or been treated for psychiatric illness, your attitude may be colored by that experience. If everything seemed to go well in the care that was received, you may not be so fearful, but you still might have worries that there could be some kind of genetic or familial transmission of vulnerability to psychiatric illness onto you. If you suffered a great deal because of your family member's psychiatric illness, or if the treatment the relative received did not seem successful or was negative, you may not have much faith in the value of psychiatric treatment.

Also, if there has been psychiatric illness in your family, you may have felt firsthand the stigma in our society toward people who live with mental illness. In that case, even if you are going to a psychiatrist only for marital therapy, you may still fear that you are going to be labeled in some way or that, because there is psychiatric illness in your family, you will be blamed for the bulk of the marital distress. Although these fears are irrational, many people have them nonetheless. It is a good idea to air them and receive reassurance from your therapist.

Issues Concerning Gender

Should We Choose a Male or a Female Therapist?

This is a good question, especially in the gender-conscious era in which we live. From a professional point of view, it doesn't matter whether your therapist is male or female. I would suggest, however, that you give this some thought and by all means discuss it with each other. You might find that you do actually have a preference, or, if not, you might at least uncover some gender-related ideas or expectations of a male versus a female therapist. If you had a previous unsatisfactory experience with a particular therapist whom you found ineffective or aggressive or with whom your spouse had a negative experience, this could affect your thinking regarding the gender of your new therapist.

A good marital therapist will understand and be sensitive to *both* men and women and will have an appreciation for your experience and your partner's experience in your marriage. In fact, you will notice immediately, or certainly within a few visits, whether you and your spouse are being understood and respected for your differing feelings, attitudes, and ways of being toward each other. I would suggest that you talk to your therapist immediately if you sense that he or she is siding with you or with your spouse. When you do this, your therapist should respond to your question or comment comfortably and nondefensively.

What do you do if you and your spouse disagree on whether to see a man or a woman? One solution is to simply flip a coin. That is probably the fairest way to do it, all other variables being equal. It is generally not a good idea to give in to your spouse's preference unless you can face this with equanimity and maturity. To give in and behave negatively from the beginning is self-defeating and a waste of time and money. What seems like a gender issue, however, may not be. It may be more characteristic of the individual's personality. Here is an example of what I mean:

Tom and Mary

Tom and Mary, both cabdrivers, brought up the issue of gender at the very beginning of their first visit with me. Mary stated that she wasn't at all comfortable coming to see me because I was a man. She stated, "I'm only here because Tom refuses to see a woman." Tom responded with "Mary is absolutely right. Our last counselor was a woman, and she was one of those man-hating feminists."

I asked both Tom and Mary to explain. Mary described their previous therapist as someone who was not a man-hating feminist but someone who believed very strongly in men and women having equal rights and responsibilities in marriage. "When she told Tom that it was only fair that he help me with the housework, he hit the roof. He told her that he worked hard enough driving all day and that he did enough work out in the yard to make up for the work I did in the home. They got into a huge argument about it and Tom stormed out of the office." Tom added, "That's more or less the way it was, but there was more to it than that. She said I was a chauvinist and that got my back up. I work with women all day long, and I don't think I'm as much of a Neanderthal as the counselor seemed to think I was."

Mary went on to explain why she was reticent to see a male therapist. "I was married once before and my husband was an alcoholic. We went to see a social worker and he told me that he would become an alcoholic too if he had to 'listen to my nagging day after day after day.' I got really angry at him; in fact, I swore at him. Then he said, 'See, that proves my point! You really are one tough woman.'"

I listened very carefully to both Tom and Mary and what they had to say about their previous therapy. Their perception of what happened was what was really most important to me. How much was gender, I don't know. In my therapy with the two of them, I found each to be excitable and provocative from time to time. I tried my best to remain calm and not to take any of their cracks personally. I remained very neutral and tried to respect each of their beliefs regarding what was "woman's work" and "man's work." With my guidance they were able to negotiate what *they* believed was a fair division of jobs around the house. Overall they did very well, and after six visits they were feeling a lot better about their marriage and were communicating much more effectively.

Since the resurgence of the women's movement in the late 1960s, there have been phenomenal changes in gender roles in our society. This has influenced the study and training of today's marital therapists and it is considered essential because of the numerous gender issues that occur in the everyday lives of men and women. Many of these factors underlie the complaints and problems that people bring to their therapists. Some examples of clinical situations with gender-related underpinnings are battered wives and battering husbands, sexual abuse, men who rape, alcoholism, workaholism, depressed homemakers, abandoned wives and husbands, custody battles, and unpaid child support payments. These are some of the types of problems that you and your spouse may be confronting. The more skill that your therapist has with these problems, the easier it will be for all of you to work together and to solve these marital difficulties. And the more your therapist is familiar with community resources for these problems, the better.

Your Gender

It's true that men are more reluctant to go for therapy than women. That said, many men are quite happy to continue in marital therapy once they get through the first visit. If that initial visit goes well, and the man's anxiety has been allayed, he will likely feel much more relaxed about continuing in treatment.

The most common reasons that men feel reticent to go for marital therapy are variants of what I have mentioned so far: a need for privacy ("I'm not going to air my dirty laundry in public"), self-reliance ("We don't need to see a therapist. We can handle our problems ourselves. I've been doing it all my life"), and previous experience with a therapist that was negative ("I went to see a therapist with my first wife. A lot of good that did. She dumped me."). For many men, going for marital therapy is a sign of weakness; it is not "macho." It is the antithesis of the traditional male role.

Marital therapy can be scary, if not terrifying, for men because its basic premise has to do with communication, and communication about feelings, the thought of which may be overwhelming and intimidating. Because men are used to communicating in a much more condensed, intellectualized, and practical way, the idea of being in a situation charged with feeling and that feels somewhat ambiguous will seem quite foreign.

Finally, many men approach marital therapy fearing that they will be "one down." They have a mind-set that there is a winner and a loser. They fear that they will be the loser because of their perception that their wife will be in a setting with another person (the therapist) who speaks her language. It's a feeling of being "the odd man out." This is exemplified in the words of one man, describing his previous experience in therapy with his first wife:

> When my former wife and I went into marital therapy, I really felt like a misfit. Although the therapist was a man, he and my wife, a psychologist, clearly had a common bond. As an engineer I felt completely out to lunch. They both kept telling me that I was too much in my head and that I was trying to solve our marital problems using engineering principles. It was pretty tough for me, and after a few visits I refused to go back. So far, this feels a bit different here, but I've got to warn you, Dr. Myers, I've really got my guard up.

If you and your therapist are of the same sex, you can expect a type of identification that is relatively straightforward and easy to understand. The therapist will be tuned in to gender issues, however, and you should not feel that your therapist is siding with you against your spouse. If you and your therapist are of the opposite sex, you should still feel that he or she understands you, and the therapist may be trying even harder to understand your feelings and your frustrations in your marriage. I emphasize this point because of the power dynamics in marriage and in marital therapy. Whenever a therapist sees a heterosexual couple, there are always two people in the room of one sex and one person of the opposite sex. The "singleton" should never feel disadvantaged, marginalized, ganged-up on, or scapegoated. If that feeling exists, it must be discussed openly in the course of treatment.

Other Concerns

If your spouse is a therapist (of any discipline), he or she may be reluctant to go for help because of embarrassment, feelings of failure, or lack of faith in the process of therapy (despite being a therapist). You may get the sense that your spouse is minimizing your distress as a couple. Just because someone is a therapist does not mean that this person has all the answers to life's bumpy road. Furthermore, it is possible to be a very successful and highly respected therapist with a wonderful ability to help others and still have problems yourself. All human beings can benefit from the watchful eye, and sense of support, that can only come from someone outside your situation.

A final concern, and one that is quite common in the cultural mosaic of our contemporary world, is to what degree our cultural, racial, ethnic, or religious background influences our attitudes toward marital therapy. Some people easily recognize the need for and expected benefits of professional help. Others, because of familial privacy or cultural pride, would never consider seeing a therapist about their marriage. Hence, intermarried couples sometimes have difficulty going to see someone for treatment.

TWELVE
The Outcome
Expectations and Reality

Your Expectations of Therapy

The Therapist

It is best to view your marital therapist as a trained professional who is there to offer you help as a consultant and as an assistant. Even though the entire process of marital therapy begins with a consultation visit or two, your therapist will be continuing to function in a consultative capacity throughout the course of your work together. In other words, your therapist will be assessing your marriage continually while assisting the two of you from visit to visit.

You will notice that your therapist will attempt to identify your specific areas of conflict and try to determine how each of you contributes to these conflicts. One of the primary goals of psychotherapy, including marital therapy, is to increase your understanding. By making these underlying dynamics more obvious and visible to the two of you, your therapist helps you attain a clearer understanding of your issues. Further, your marital therapist should be able to help the two of you work toward getting rid of habitual and ineffectual communication patterns as well as learn new ways of communicating with each other. The environment for this process should be an encouraging and facilitating one that begins in the office but allows the two of you to still go on with your daily lives.

No matter what the theoretical orientation of your therapist, most will concentrate on your current issues and problems, the ones that are causing the two of you distress. This will likely feel most appropriate to both of you and will yield the most change. However, there may be some old issues standing in the way of progress. Therefore, it will be necessary for your therapist to draw connections between your present behavior, values, and attitudes and the past. The purpose is to help you understand and explain why each of you acts and reacts the way you do. It is only with this kind of emotional and intellectual knowledge that you can begin to work at changing. And if change is not possible, at least you and your spouse can work toward accepting your situation for what it is.

You and your spouse should expect a safe, mutually respectful, and nonjudgmental relationship with your marital therapist. You may not always feel it to the same degree or at the same time, but this type of relationship is fundamental and is the foundation of effective therapy. Remember that being nonjudgmental is not the same as being unfeeling, underactive, passive, or detached. At times you might even find your therapist quite direct and even confrontational. But it is possible to be this way in a firm yet kind and nonmoralistic way. You both should feel that your therapist has your best interests at heart.

The Therapy Experience

Although each therapist has a unique style of marital therapy, let me briefly describe my approach with the hope that I can allay some of the anxiety that most couples experience when first coming to therapy.

Your first visit. In the first interview I delineate your complaints and attempt to understand how each of you defines the problems. I then ask if you both agree with my assessment. I also want to know how long you have had these concerns, if they are affecting your mental health, and how these problems manifest themselves in your day-to-day relationship. For example, do you fight a lot, is there tension, or are you afraid to talk or to confront each other? Next, I want to know if you have some ideas about the factors contributing to the surface complaints. Also in the first visit, I want to know if the two of you have had any previous marital therapy and, if so, how each of you felt about that experience.

If you and your spouse have separated before, I need to know about the circumstances, how long the two of you were actually apart, how that felt, and the events and feelings surrounding your reconciliation. I am especially interested in knowing whether you felt your problems were resolved and if you feel that the current difficulties are new or a reactivation or continuation of the old problems. I will also want to know if you are hopeful about marital therapy being helpful or whether you sense another separation looming on the horizon.

It's important for me to have a sense of what the two of you have in common, your shared interests, activities, recreational pursuits, culture, sports, and children. Do you have separate interests and, if so, what is the balance in your relationship between doing things on your own (or with friends) or together as a couple?

I will try to get a sense of how committed you each feel to your marriage. If you don't feel very committed, you are not alone. Many couples are conscious of the fact that they are barely hanging on and do not feel they really want the marriage to continue. It's also important for me to gauge how committed each of you is to the therapy process. But once again, if you are not equally committed, do not worry. It is hard to be committed to "working on your marriage" when you're uncertain whether you wish to remain married. Most marital therapists are quite willing to take one visit at a time with couples who are uncertain about their future together.

If there is still time remaining in the first visit, I will begin to ask about the history of your relationship. How did the two of you meet? How was your courtship? How long was it? Did any problems arise during the courtship? Did you live together before you got married? If so, how was that period? How was your early sexual experience together? Any problems in this area? Has there been any change in your sexual pattern as your relationship has evolved? If there have been some changes in your lovemaking, did they seem related to other problems that you are having or external stresses in your lives? In the first visit, I would not go into detailed questions concerning your sexual relationship unless it seemed appropriate.

The next step.   The above description is a rather ambitious plan for my first visit with the two of you. The next step is a visit with each of you alone. I use these visits to learn things from each of you about your early developmental years, your family, your adolescence and young adulthood, and any previous serious relationships or marriages. I also like to take a general medical history, during which I can ask about your physical health, allergies, medications, and any connection between your physical health and your mental health. If you have had psychiatric illness before and have seen a psychiatrist, I can ask you about this in the privacy of your individual visit with me. These individual visits are solely for my purposes. They enable me to get to know each of you in much more depth and detail. They are completely confidential, and I do not discuss what I learn in these individual visits with your spouse or with the two of you when we again sit down together.

Most couples find the individual visits very helpful. It gives each of you an opportunity to be candid about matters that may be difficult to talk about, even if you have shared them with each other, when your spouse is present. It also gives each of you a chance to tell me about any secrets you feel are important in terms of my understanding you and the difficulties you had before or are having now in your marriage.

Not all marital therapists will want to see each of you alone. In fact, some refuse to do so. They do not want to know any secrets. On the other hand, as a physician, I am used to "a head full of secrets." Patients have confided in me since I was a medical student, and I believe this is part of the doctor-patient covenant. People should have an opportunity to confide in their doctor about anything that has caused or is causing them distress. Some examples of secrets that you might feel the need to discuss would be an undisclosed previous marriage, a pregnancy you have not told your husband about, an abortion or abortions, previous psychiatric treatment, sexual abuse, a homosexual experience at some earlier time in your life, a period of "promiscuity," a criminal record, and an extramarital affair.

In my individual visit you might find that I am interested in selective details about your personal and family history. I like to obtain some sense of your ability to cope with your frustrations, how you adapt to stress, and how you handle disappointments. I also want to assess your level of self-esteem, self-confidence, and overall maturity for your chronological age. It is important to me to get some sense of your independence and interdependence. My understanding of your ability to love and your capacity for love is also part of my assessment, as are your respective abilities to give support to each other and to accept support from each other.

The above is a short summary to give you an idea of what might happen in your early visits with a marital therapist. Although all therapists work somewhat differently according to their training, their experience, and their general professional style, most therapists approach and assess couples with quite a broad perspective. Certain elements of your "story" will be focused on more than others. In other words, certain elements will be much more important to your therapist than others, and if there's not much time, there may be some prioritizing of issues. You and your spouse, of course, have very unique backgrounds, and what your therapist emphasizes might be quite different from what he or she emphasizes with your spouse. In this way, your therapist will be able to determine the ways in which the two of you complement each other and the ways in which you don't. The more you can tell your therapist about yourself and what makes you tick, the more your therapy should be rewarding and helpful. This richness in detail moves your marital therapy away from a superficial analysis by your therapist and "counseling" onto a deeper plane.

What's Supposed to Happen?

The object of therapy, of course, is for the two of you to feel better. The route to this may be somewhat circuitous; you should definitely feel a lot clearer about yourself, your spouse, and your marriage, if therapy is helping. This process may be slow at times and also painful because marital therapy involves looking at things that haven't made any sense to you before or facing things that you have been pushing away for some time.

Some people have the mistaken notion that marital therapy causes couples to separate. Marital therapy can't *make* you separate. Those couples who do separate in the midst of therapy were already on their way to separation before their therapy started. The therapy has merely confirmed that their relationship is in serious trouble and that separation is necessary or inevitable. Overall, the number of people who do separate with marital therapy is quite small compared with the number who *fear* separation.

Once you have established a rapport and feel comfortable with your therapist, you should be able to open up and talk about your feelings in therapy. You can express feelings about your relationship and also talk directly to your spouse in the therapy session. In fact, you may find your therapist deliberately trying to get you to talk about the appropriate feelings you should be experiencing when a particular subject is being discussed. This mobilization is especially critical if you have unconscious feelings about something (feelings of which you aren't aware) or if there are feelings that are hiding behind certain types of behavior on your part that are upsetting your spouse. Airing these feelings in the therapy session will make you feel better, less tense, and will improve understanding between you and your spouse.

If you are a person who has no difficulty facing feelings or at times feels actually overwhelmed by feelings (especially negative feelings), your therapist will try to help you contain these strong emotions. This will not be done in a controlling or suppressive way but in a way that will make you, and your spouse, feel more comfortable. Your therapist may attempt to slow things down a bit in the sessions and to help both of you be still and listen to each other.

What else can you expect in marital therapy? Well, if you and your spouse are in the midst of a very serious crisis and this is what brings you to marital therapy, you should be able to count on your therapist until the worst is over and you have begun to see your way clearly again. An example of this might be a situation in which your partner just told you that he or she is having an affair and you are feeling hurt, angry, and confused.

What do I mean by "counting on" your therapist? I mean this quite literally—you should be able to lean on that person, seek advice, and even take comfort or solace from your therapist. In these early days or weeks you are often not yourself. You have regressed and you may feel anxious and panicky, confused, indecisive, furious, despondent, in and out of control, and disorganized. Further, you may not trust your own judgment. A seasoned therapist will understand this and will respond warmly and with interest and concern. If you're also feeling symptomatic—not sleeping well, eating poorly, having physical pain, not working efficiently—your therapist might suggest a more thorough assessment and possibly medication. Your therapist may refer you to your primary care physician and possibly a psychiatrist. At any rate, no major life decision should be made until you begin to feel better again and regain your usual level of function, purpose, order, self-control, and mood stability.

He Says, She Says . . .

He says: "I wish she wouldn't get so emotional. When we discuss things or when she's angry, she gets hysterical."

She says: "Why can't he be a better listener? When I talk about my day, he either fades out or starts giving me advice."

Men who make statements like this are really saying that they like to discuss things in a calm and cool manner with little feeling being expressed. When their wives cry, some men get angry because they don't trust the tears, or they begin to feel guilty, or they find the crying time-consuming when they want the discussion over and done with. Many don't realize that crying is physiological—a physical accompaniment to feelings of sadness, frustration, anger, or hurt.

And it does hurt to know that the person who supposedly loves you is not listening or doesn't seem interested in what you have to say. Some of this might be due to different communication styles. Men usually concentrate on one thing at a time, so if a woman tries to talk when her husband has his mind on something else, he may have trouble giving her his full attention. And many men instinctively offer advice in an effort to solve the problem, when all their wives want is to talk about their feelings and be listened to. Advice, in fact, may make a woman feel cut off and dismissed.

If your marital problem is of long duration and simply seems to be chugging along without a crisis, a marital therapist should be able to help the two of you begin to talk again, to communicate more effectively, to make decisions together, and to feel more intimate together (both sexually and nonsexually). Just making the decision to go to see someone for your marriage helps tremendously. It means that each of you cares enough about the other, about your marriage, and about your family to want to do your best to try to improve things and, if at all possible, to preserve your marriage. You are basically making a commitment to each other to try—and for many people that is the most they can promise each other, in all good faith.

Young couples who are in their early years together and couples who are somewhat isolated from their friends and family can feel very reassured by their marital therapist. They often simply need a reassurance that their troubles are quite common, probably transient, and easily remediable.

You should come away from therapy with a new perspective on your marriage, how serious your problems are, and which are more pressing. This perspective may actually be quite subtle and hard to put into words, but it is a common corollary of marital therapy. It is expressed in statements like this:

> I'm not exactly sure what worked in our therapy with Dr. Green. I know that he made some suggestions and pointed out things that each of us was doing that needed work, but there was something else going on. There was something about his manner that was very, very reassuring, that gave us hope, that made us feel that we would get through this difficult time, that our problems were manageable. And he got us laughing again. We were even able to laugh at some of our difficulties that we had both viewed so ominously before we went to see him.

If your problems are very serious, or more serious than they originally seemed to be, your therapist should be able to make a commitment to assist you as much as possible. No matter how demoralized you both may feel, you should begin to feel more optimistic about things changing in your marriage. If your conflict is so serious that separation seems the only logical answer, you should feel that your therapist is genuinely concerned and is there to assist and support each of you through that process, as well as the children.

How Do You Know
if Therapy Is Working?

The answer to this question is easy. You should be able to feel some change in yourself in as few as four to six visits (or even sooner, depending on how poorly you've been feeling or how long you've been experiencing marital difficulty). What do I mean by change? You should feel a bit happier, you should have fewer symptoms of distress, you should feel less angry or less anxious, or less sad and more hopeful. Your partner should feel somewhat better as well, but don't expect that you both will feel the same way at the same time. Marital therapy visits vary tremendously in their power and how they affect each of you. You may find that some visits feel much more productive than others, and you will leave the therapy hour feeling quite elated and hopeful. Other visits may not feel nearly as productive or beneficial. At times like that, you may wonder if you're making any progress at all.

What are some of the signs that you can look for in yourself that will give you a feeling of change? Your communication with each other should flow more easily. This could mean that you begin to communicate in a way that is novel and quite exciting. Or change could mean that you and your spouse are communicating like you used to, and this will be a relief too. Another point is that you should be able to discuss sensitive subjects with each other more easily. You may find that you are opening up more and talking about matters that had been frightening for you in the past or that you are listening more attentively to your spouse. You may be more open to learning new things about each other, and you may be setting aside more time together.

If your way of talking with each other had been cruel, stylized, stiff, or intellectualized, you may note now that you and your partner are talking more intimately and with more feeling. If your dialogue with each other had been extremely volatile, with a lot of high emotion, you may find yourselves speaking in a much more relaxed and calm manner. If your communication previously seemed to make each of you defensive and hostile, you should now be able to talk to each other with more trust and less feeling of being attacked or being on the attack.

Something else you might note is that your ability to identify your issues has become clearer. Likewise, your decision making should be easier. There should be fewer misunderstandings, less mind reading, less preemptive thinking about your spouse, and just a more comfortable sense of knowing where you stand with each other.

If you and your spouse had been agonizing over whether to remain together, and your marriage has been in serious trouble, a decision one way or the other should be easier after a few visits with your marital therapist. It is very common to feel hopeless about your marriage when you begin therapy. In fact, you may have had a feeling like this: "Living like this is driving me crazy and making me very despondent. Unless something changes, I'm not sure if I can go on. I will have to leave." For most couples in marital therapy, things do indeed change.

For some couples, however, things do not turn around. What becomes clear after a few visits with your marital therapist is that your uncertain decision to separate crystallizes, and you realize that you must proceed with living apart. You will probably experience a sense of relief with this realization; that is, you have come to a decision to separate, finally, after so many months or years of agonizing.

I suggest that you both have a frank talk with your therapist if you don't feel any change or if you feel a worsening of your situation after you have a few therapy visits. In fact, I suggest that you have this discussion even if only one of you feels this way. What is important is that you express these feelings and have some kind of clarification or validation of your feelings in the therapeutic meeting. Feeling that there has been no change could be part of a problem with your expectations. You may be expecting change to occur too quickly, given the duration of your marital difficulty and the number of appointments that you have had with your therapist. In other words, you are expecting major change when only minor change in your situation is realistic at that point. Your therapist will explore these expectations with you in such a way that you feel understood. His or her manner should be open and respectful, and you should experience a sense of relief that you are not wasting your time in therapy. After a discussion like that, you should feel good about continuing in therapy and that this decision is entirely your own or yours as a couple; that is, you have not been forced, pushed, manipulated, or shamed by your therapist into continuing therapy.

One important thing to note: If you feel that things are getting worse, this could be an indication that things are actually getting better and that the therapy is working. More specifically, issues that have been pushed away and relegated to "the back burner" are now being felt at the surface, are being talked about, and are generating symptoms in one or both of you. In this regard, your therapist should be helpful in explaining this to you in a way that makes sense and is reassuring. It is indeed true that some couples feel worse before they feel better. What is characteristic, though, is that this phenomenon should fluctuate from day to day or week to week; a feeling of worsening should not persist without relief for days or weeks on end. Your therapist should be curious about and monitor these feelings carefully with the two of you at each visit. Your worry about them should become your therapist's concern. Your therapist may even suggest a change of format (by seeing each of you on your own for a few visits), a change in the frequency or timing of your appointments, or even a second opinion from an experienced marital therapist colleague.

There is no reason to stay in therapy with someone who is not meeting your needs. Both you and your spouse should feel that your therapist has your best interests at heart, is being supportive, and is trying to assist the two of you as you negotiate your way clear of your problems. Remember that you are paying for a professional service and therefore you have a right to expect certain things of your therapist. And you can always decide to see someone else.

I can't emphasize enough how important it is to discuss openly your expectations of therapy with your therapist, especially those you feel are not being met. I believe that most adults approach marital therapy with realistic expectations and know that there are no miracles. But still, it is not always easy to determine how much change can be expected or achieved. As a consumer of a service, you can't help but feel disappointed in yourselves or your therapist if the changes that you are making are very slow, painful, frightening, or not very great.

Only by talking about these issues with your therapist will you be able to have your questions answered—questions that connect with feelings of disappointment and frustration. Ask your therapist: "Are our expectations too high? Are we working hard enough in therapy? How common is it to feel this let down, and if so, can you explain that to us? Is it possible that you are not the right therapist for us, and we should look around?" These are all very important and very legitimate questions.

Finally, if you and your spouse are feeling better and are ready to end therapy, find out if your therapist is open to seeing the two of you in the future, should problems arise. The fact that your therapist will be available and, further, that you don't have to start all over again with someone new can be very reassuring. In some marriages, problems wax and wane, or stress can become overwhelming and cause a lot of upset. One or two sessions with a therapist who knows you can help.

The Question of
Individual Therapy

In certain cases your therapist might suggest individual treatment for one or both of you. If he or she carefully explains the rationale for this suggestion, the proposal should make sense and be easy to accept. You shouldn't feel like the therapist is taking sides, or that you are being singled out and have more problems than your spouse, or that you are the entire problem in your relationship.

It is a different matter if you are interested in exploring individual therapy yourself, for this means that you have some insight into your problems and are open to receiving some professional help. It could also mean that you feel "stuck" in your marriage because of some individual conflict or problem from your past that you believe needs resolution before you can communicate clearly in your relationship or move forward with your partner. It is much easier to accept the notion of individual therapy if the wish, desire, and motivation come from within you—in other words, if this is an autonomous wish that is completely by your choice.

There can be many benefits, including improved feelings about yourself, associated with individual therapy. Despite the changing roles of women and men over the past decades, there is still a gender gap in terms of interest in and willingness to explore individual psychotherapy. More women than men are interested in individual therapy. However, this discrepancy is less than it once was, as men increasingly see the benefit of individual therapy instead of seeing it as a sign of weakness or dependency.

For many people, seeing a therapist for marital problems is easier and less threatening than going for individual treatment. In some circles it is more socially acceptable to be in "marital counseling" with your husband or wife than it is to be in "therapy." As a doctor, I have had many experiences with couples who prefer to see me as a "counselor" rather than as a psychiatrist. Seeing a psychiatrist conjures up images of mental illness, whereas seeing a counselor for relationship difficulties seems less serious, less dysfunctional, less sick. It's OK to have marital problems, but it's not OK to have personal problems.

For many couples, seeing a therapist for their relationship is the ticket of admission into individual therapy. For most of us in relationships, especially something as serious as marriage, the act of facing marital tension and unhappiness is the first time that we are forced to take a hard, cold look at ourselves. This can be jarring, frightening, humbling, and exciting. Our personal weaknesses and fears stand out in bold relief when they are identified and voiced by our partner. Even if we are aware of our conflicts or personal difficulties earlier in life, we might have been very successful in pushing them away, shrugging them off, or channeling them into individual pursuits. These kinds of coping mechanisms are not always available to us when involved in a serious relationship that requires time spent together, sharing thoughts and feelings, honesty, and maturity.

You may actually find yourself filled with anticipation, if not excitement, about the prospect of individual therapy. If you've had some therapy in the past and found it helpful, then you may certainly have this kind of emotion. However, even if you have never received any individual therapy but have considered it, you may see this option as an opportunity.

APPENDIX

Where to Go for Help

Self-Help Groups

National Depressive and Manic-Depressive Association (NDMDA)
730 North Franklin Street, Suite 501
Chicago, IL 60610
Telephone: (312) 642-0049
Fax: (312) 642-7243

D/ART Program (Depression/Awareness, Recognition and Treatment)
National Institute of Mental Health
Room 10C-03
5600 Fishers Lane
Rockville, MD 20857
Telephone: (301) 443-3720
Fax: (301) 443-4045

Panic Disorder Education Program
National Institute of Mental Health
Parklawn Building, Room 799
5600 Fishers Lane
Rockville, MD 20857
Telephone: (800) 64-PANIC (647-2642)

National Alliance for the Mentally Ill (NAMI)
200 North Glebe Road
Suite 1015
Arlington, VA 22203-3754
Telephone: (703) 524-7600, (800) 950-NAMI
Fax: (703) 524-9094

National Mental Health Association
1021 Prince Street
Alexandria, VA 22314
Telephone: (703) 684-7722
Fax: (703) 684-5968

Recovery, Incorporated (Association of Nervous and Former Mental Patients)
802 North Dearborn Street
Chicago, IL 60610
Telephone: (312) 337-5661
Fax: (312) 337-5756

National Associations for Marriage Therapists

National Association for Marriage and Family Therapy

American Family Therapy Association

American Counseling Association

American Association of Sex Educators, Counselors, and Therapists

American Association of Pastoral Counselors

American Psychological Association

National Association of Social Workers

American Orthopsychiatric Association

American Psychiatric Association

Suggested Readings

Beattie M: Codependent No More: How to Stop Controlling Others and Start Caring for Yourself. New York, HarperCollins, 1987

Beck A: Love Is Never Enough: How Couples Can Overcome Misunderstandings, Resolve Conflicts, and Solve Relationship Problems Through Cognitive Therapy. New York, Harper & Row, 1988

Benedek EP, Brown CF: How to Help Your Child Overcome Your Divorce. Washington, DC, American Psychiatric Press, 1995

Burns DD: Feeling Good: The New Mood Therapy. New York, William Morrow, 1980

Covington S, Beckett L: Leaving the Enchanted Forest: The Path From Relationship Addiction to Intimacy. San Francisco, CA, Harper, 1988

Cronkite K: On the Edge of Darkness: Conversations About Conquering Depression. New York, Bantam Doubleday Dell, 1994

Depaulo JR, Ablow KR: How to Cope With Depression: A Companion Guide for You and Your Family. New York, McGraw-Hill, 1989

From Survival to Recovery: Growing Up in an Alcoholic Home. New York, Alanon Family Groups Headquarters, 1994

Greist JH, Jefferson JW: Depression and Its Treatment, Revised Edition. Washington, DC, American Psychiatric Press, 1992

Greist JH, Jefferson JW, Marks IM: Anxiety and Its Treatment: Help Is Available. Washington, DC, American Psychiatric Press, 1986

Hochschild A: The Time Bind: When Work Becomes Home and Home Becomes Work. New York, Metropolitan Books/Henry Holt & Company, 1997

Jamison KR: An Unquiet Mind: A Memoir of Moods and Madness. New York, Alfred A. Knopf, 1995

Mooney A, Eisenberg A, Eisenberg H, et al: The Recovery Book. New York, Houghton Mifflin, 1992

"Post-Traumatic Stress Disorder," published by the American Psychiatric Association, 1400 K Street, NW, Washington, DC 20005 (Free)

"Post-Traumatic Stress Disorder," published by the Anxiety Disorders Association of America, 6000 Executive Blvd., No 513, Rockville, MD 20852 ($2.50)

Ross J: Triumph Over Fear. New York, Bantam Books, 1995

Scarf M: Intimate Partners: Patterns in Love and Marriage. New York, Random House, 1987

Seigel M, Brimsman J, Weinshel M: Surviving an Eating Disorder. New York, Harper & Row, 1988

Sherman RT, Thompson RA: Bulimia: A Guide for Family and Friends. San Diego, CA, Lexington Books, 1990

Styron W: Darkness Visible: A Memoir of Madness. New York, Random House, 1990

Tannen D: You Just Don't Understand: Women and Men in Conversation. New York, William Morrow, 1990

Weiner-Davis M: Divorce Busting: A Revolutionary and Rapid Program for Staying Together. New York, Summit Books, 1992

Index